Addiction: Why They Use

A Handbook for Anyone Who Loves an

Alcoholic or Addict

Emmanuel S. John

Baltimore
2012

Addiction: Why They Use
(A Handbook for Anyone Who Loves an Alcoholic or Addict)
2nd Edition
Copyright © 2012 by Emmanuel S. John

ISBN 978-0-9851898-0-8

Printed in the USA

This book is dedicated to my spiritual mother and guide
Joyce Luciano
God bless her beautiful soul.

To my father,
Raymond John, killed by addiction.

This book is also dedicated to all those people
who suffer needlessly at the hand of a twisted disease,
and to every alcoholic and addict who has refused to
sell out to that disease.

Table of Contents

PART I
The Journey Begins

PART II
HOW & WHY

PART III
Addiction, and Mental Illness

PART IV
Denial

PART V
STRESS: Why They Use and Use and Use

PART VI
Enabling

PART VII
Stumbling Block to Stepping Stones

Introduction

I am happy that you have made the choice to increase your awareness about substance addiction by examining this book. You will be glad you did. This book has been written with a very specific, very clear purpose: that purpose is to increase individual awareness of the "nature" of addiction in our society. My goal is to clearly explain what it truly means to be emotionally addicted as well as how that emotional addiction affects the people who personally come into contact with the substance or by extension the addict/alcoholic. This book is a handbook for anyone who loves someone who is addicted.

The information contained in the following pages will undoubtedly improve your perspective of the ills that are "Addiction." The war we wage against substance abuse and dependency will never change until we understand both the enemy and the battlefield. If we truly want things to change we must understand both the physiological and psychological-emotional natures of the disease. Understanding only half the problem will only perpetuate the problem. The lack of a comprehensive understanding of the disease of addiction only results in more emotional pain for those of us who love or have loved an addict/alcoholic.

This book is not a technical manual on addiction nor is it a scientific examination of the physiological effects of addiction: Those topics have been investigated with little benefit beyond more drugs to treat a drug problem. Instead, this book is an examination of the emotional side of addiction; the root causes of the problem. By writing this book this author hopes to reduce the pain endured by those who have been affected by substance use and abuse. If it is technical and scientific data that you desire then I encourage you to seek out my counter parts in the addiction research field at the National Institute of Drug Abuse (www.nida.gov.)

While some physiological aspects will be discussed in this book the major focus will be on how the emotional aspects of addiction plague both the user and their significant family members. This book is the culmination of more than 25 years of deeply devoted examination of the still using, the chronic relapser, the newly abstinent and those persons with long-term, sustained recovery of up to 40 years or more. We will also examine the personal practices of people who have since recovered from their addiction and examine those traits, which have proven most successful.

As a clinical professional I have dedicated my life to helping people get past their need to use and to heal the pain resulting from substance use for both the user and their loved ones. My goal has always been to help my clients and their families' gain/regain healthier emotional lives. An important personal goal of mine has been to return addictive families to a more normal, healthier state of functioning. Since I can't possibly meet with you all personally I've written this book to share with you my understanding and our successes.

In the following pages I will refer to addiction, alcoholism, substance abuse and substance dependency. For our purposes and for the majority of the topics discussed the terms are fairly interchangeable but it should be noted that there are clinical differences that exist. These variances will be identified when necessary. The term addict does not exclusively refer to the illicit drug user but to the abuser of alcohol and prescription drugs as well.

Almost all abstinence based addiction treatment in this country has evolved from the practices developed in the past 100 years. For reasons of clarity the book begins with a specific focus on the history of how alcoholism (addiction to alcohol) has been viewed and treated. This does not suggest that the problem of addiction is anything new. There are references to addiction as far back as the Book of Solomon in the Bible. For practical reasons we will focus mainly on the trends of the past 100 years, as they are much more germane to our primary goal, which is again to understand the emotional problems of addiction. Because we are focusing on the emotional aspects of addiction there is little difference in the emotional torture experienced by today's users or by the users of 100 or even 2000 years ago, regardless of their drug of choice.

About the Author

Having worked and volunteered in the field of addiction for more than 25 years, I have learned several basic truths about addiction that I would like to share with you. I share these truths with the hope of lessening the torment you may be experiencing because of this dreadful disease. This book has been written with the primary goal of lessening the pains of addiction for you: for the addict, the addicted's family and all the other primary or significant figures in the addicted's life. Its idea is simple; we lessen the pain by understanding and depersonalizing the nature of the illness.

I am a clinical professional. I began my work with addicts back in the glory days of the 28-day treatment program when insurance companies paid for a somewhat more practical level of care. (It should be noted that 28 days is not a clinically significant number, it was an insurance company payment limitation. There are some addicted people that require as much as a year of treatment in a structured program to overcome their malady.)

I have worked in nearly all the abstinence based modalities of drug treatment including, long term inpatient (more than 28 days), 28 days treatment programs, forensic/jail based programs, Intensive Outpatient Programs (IOP), non-intensive Out Patient Treatment Programs (often referred to as drug counseling,) early intervention and even in prevention programs working with elementary school children in the 3rd, 4th and 5th grades. In addition to working with addicts directly, I have worked extensively with the family members and the loved ones of addicts regardless of their ages. In order to share the awareness that I have attained with the greatest number of people, I have also designed and conducted numerous professional trainings on this subject to help other addiction professionals become more effective care givers.

In regards to diversity, I consider myself extremely fortunate to have had a vast amount of exposure to different cultural groups. I worked for nearly 7 years in the Baltimore City Public School system, some integrated but most predominantly African American. Never shying away from a challenge I have often entered some of the toughest schools in a city full of "tough" schools, sometimes when other professionals could no longer persevere. During this time I conducted one of the longest running drug dealers groups in the city.

I later spent 4 years working with Jewish people of all devotional levels from the totally unconnected to the most Orthodox of Orthodox families. Remember, addiction is a disease. Being a disease it affects a portion of the population regardless of religious affiliation, family nurturing, socioeconomic level, or functioning.

After I attained my clinical education I decided to enter into a program at the University of Maryland for a degree in "Instructional Systems Development." While there, I did recovery specific research and attained more insight into educational design. This allowed me to increase the effectiveness of substance abuse education so that more people can be better informed about this serious illness. I would love to receive your feedback once you have read this book (www.whytheyuse.com)(whytheyuse@gmail.com) (addictioninthefamily.com)

Part I

The Journey Begins

Getting to the Truth

The most basic of all truths about addiction is; addiction hurts. It hurts not only the addicted, but by extension all those persons who have to relate to and/or are reliant upon the addicted. It has been my experience that the significant others of addicts (this includes all those who are in regular contact with the addict) often suffer more than the addict as they do not have the luxury of chemical escape from the reality of the situation.

We will examine this pain-full issue of addiction on several levels. First, we will define addiction through the eyes of society from religious doctrines to the "modern" health care system in place today. We will do this by an examination of the views established in the United States over the past 100 years as these perceptions have most vividly colored our present understanding and misunderstanding as well. During this process we will also examine how society has defined addiction, as this most directly dictates and establishes our treatment of the addict and by extension our treatment approaches.

If what the ancient Greek existentialist said is true that; *"We are not so much bothered by things, as by our interpretation of things,"* then perhaps an insightful and unbiased view of addiction may actually serve to ease some of our duress. If the above is true then how we as a society view addiction, predicates the level of discomfort we feel as a member of that society struggling to regain manageability.

13

The War In Raging

Our first Chapter will use the history of US social perspectives on addiction and the history of addiction treatment to highlight the successes and failures of coping with and addressing the addiction problem. During the process you will inevitably notice how these perspectives have influenced your own understanding and misunderstanding of the problem. It is my hope that by bringing these truths to light you will develop for yourself, a more comprehensive understanding of the problem and the task at hand: That you will then be able to let go of the guilt and regret you may now feel.

If there was a war on drugs then we have for all intents and purposes lost that war. We have surrendered and are now living under the invading forces occupation, at their whim. If it is a war then it is a Holocaust, with millions dying around the world as a direct or indirect result. While we may have won the battle of treatment availability we have lost the war on importation and recreation. Many of us do not even know who the real enemy is.

General Patten said; "I have seen the enemy and he is us." Biblical references tell us to "Know thy enemy." Sounds pretty serious doesn't it? Is there really anyone who believes we have won or are winning? Seriously? Is there a cohesive accounting of the problem under which people can join together and triumph? Is our intelligence flawed?

What we can be sure of and all agree on is this: We are losing the war via our children's lives and their futures because we have not yet truly identified the core problems. We have not accentuated the "ills" of addiction in such a way that our youth find the risk of using a drug to be counterproductive to finding happiness and contentment. While alcohol is considered a

14

gateway drug, the use of nicotine and caffeine teach our children how to medicate emotional states. These drugs teach our children to chemically alter their state of being, rather than improve their level of insight. They learn to go for the quick fix rather than take the time and energy required to improve emotional awareness, which also fosters positive self-esteem.

When it comes to our children it is important to remember that we cannot relay a value that we ourselves do not hold. If we take the hypocrite role, our children will see right through us and discredit our future insights. They see our hypocrisy and as a result we lose our credibility. In order for us to prevent future generations from falling prey to the ignorance of the quick "FIX" we need to end that ignorance by an in-depth study of the "emotional" and "psycho-spiritual problems" which breed addiction and diminish resistance to the disease.

For far too many years now our focus regarding addiction treatment has been predicated on a failed belief that by understanding human physiology we will be able to address the emotional soul-sickness of abuse and dependence. It hasn't worked. Understanding cancer doesn't cure it; preventing cancer is the best course. Substance use is not natural. We can't put poisons and toxins in our bodies and not expect a negative result.

Think for a minute about why it is that all of the truly successful methods of overcoming addiction focus on the spiritual malady. Maybe it is because personal emotional dysfunction is the root cause of the illness. By spiritual sickness I am referring to ills of the human spirit: those of emotional outlook, self-concept, self-esteem, self-efficacy and personal self-worth.

It is possible that we may have over analyzed the problem? It's like we have been trying to cure the cancer only in its late stages instead of trying to catch it early or prevent it entirely. Unfortunately, this perspective is late for some but that doesn't mean that addiction can't be prevented or that it can't be defeated in its earlier stages with our youth and young adults.

Perhaps the solution is in treating the initial cause for use, which is to simply and quickly feel better than we do. That's right. It's that simple. People use because they want to change the way they feel. People who already feel good, content and whole, have no need to change or alter their perception because they are CONTENT with how they feel. While even the most emotionally healthy of persons can be swayed by others to experiment with drugs, these healthy minds have "faith" in their own function: They also have faith in the people and the world around them. People with a sense of self-efficacy rarely fall prey to peer-pressure and social inertias. They become leaders in a search for an alternative way to feel better, one that does not include drugs and alcohol.

The above point was not made to suggest that the solution is in any way religious. While these approaches may work for many, the human spirit does not require dogma of any kind to right itself and to return to what is natural.

This is where we start:
- Getting the chemicals out of the toxic mind is our first priority
- Mending the damage done from the drugs is our second
- Preventing further use by the installation of hope that by remaining off drugs (of all kinds) that they/we can find that contentment and happiness initially sought from the drug of choice.

As a society we are over committed to alcohol in our lives. Alcohol itself offers no sustenance for the human body or soul, yet few can imagine life without it.

Giving Treatment the Treatment
Learning from our Past

While examining each of the various treatment approaches of the past 100 years, you will undoubtedly discover how the perceived "Reason or Cause" of addiction has resulted in the treatment tactics of each of the specific methods or paradigms presented. In essence, what you will see is how over the past 100 years society has treated addiction based on what is believed to have been the cause or the reason the use started in the first place. While knowing why use started in the first place is important in regards to aspects of drug prevention, very few addicts use for the same reasons that initially compelled them to use or to continue use. While peers may have influenced their first use most addicts eventually care little about the concerns of others unless those views support continued use. (We will discuss denial in later chapters.)

Our societal approach to addressing addiction seems to be a very "Westernized" way of responding to personal struggles or difficulties. The emotional/behavioral mindset most often held by the addict is usually referred to as the seeking of "Instant Gratification." The following example may seem oversimplified but never the less it seems to be our frequent approach to finding emotional happiness and contentment in the Western World during the last century.

Consider the following; if we believed that exposure to the color blue between the ages of 7 and 9 caused a major illness we would take great pains as a society to protect our children from that color for those specific years. Perhaps we would even outlaw the use of those colors with the exception of the sky and water for which we would then develop special water dyes, contact lens or sunglasses, which could exclude that color from the light spectrum. Why? Because no one wants his or her child to acquire an illness that could have easily been prevented.

This attempt at exclusion is exactly what we have tried to do in the past when treating addiction. The approach is successful when trying to prevent addiction but apparently not for treating it. Remember Prohibition? A Constitutional amendment to treat an emotional illness! Doesn't that seem a little bizarre now? Something else that's bizarre, trying to transmit self-esteem and self-worth when we don't have it ourselves (recall the hypocrite?) Trying to get our children to delay gratification when all they see is gluttony and excess doesn't make sense either. Even more futile than that is trying to instill hope, positive self-concept, and positive regard for others into our children's hearts when we have little for ourselves or our partners. Don't think this is the case? Well then consider if hope, positive self-concept, and positive regard were present in your last lover's quarrel or when your child misbehaved.

The above points may not seem pleasant and may be hard to face but remember what we established earlier? We are at war, and war is not pleasant. There are casualties at war and our excesses, greed, and needs to feel good or right, may need to be the first sacrifices.

Unfortunately the true solution is larger than the scope of this book. During war we lose people close to us. During war we learn how to grieve for not only the losses of life, but for the loss of how we would like things to be. We learn acceptance and begin to treat the living, the survivors.

We will now begin to examine the methods used in the past for treating the casualties of the war on drugs. Those people left behind to feel the pain of a society (not a government) that has failed to address its biggest health care problem. Personally

I have not heard a word about addiction uttered in any government discussions about health care since 1996. Do you remember hearing the term "drug treatment" in 2009 while people ranted and raved about the health needs of our country? Hummmmm….. Of course not! It would have broken the bank. Imagine giving $4,000 to $20,000 to each addict per treatment attempt or episode. Multiply that by the estimated 10% of the population (30 million) that struggles with addictive issues. That is not the point of this book but leaving out one of our biggest health care problems we face should give you concern.

We Need Knowledge

What good is knowledge? Abraham Maslow said that: "Full knowledge leads to right action. Right action is impossible without full knowledge." He was suggesting that if an action is taken and it is the correct one but it was chosen outside of the full grasp of a situation that this was not right action only luck. He suggested that right action was a direct application of gained awareness. Very few people in this country ever take the time to learn about this crisis. Even recovering addicts rarely take the time to enter the term "addiction" into a search engine to gain more understanding. Somehow, addicts believe that since they have the disease they know all they need to know about it. I know of no other disease where the victim intuits some automatic knowledge of the illness because they have it.

Once again, I thank you for taking the time to read this book, by doing so you are living in the true and possibly only, solution to this problem; gaining full knowledge.

It is my belief that a true knowledge of the emotional pain associated with addiction will bring you relief. An understanding of the emotional dilemma faced by the using person will aid "significant others" in depersonalizing the addicts behavior and thereby lessening the guilt felt by loved ones who are forced to make tough, even harsh decisions for everyone involved. You can't control their lives and actions, but you can and must learn to manage your own.

By examining the following paradigms of addiction treatment we will see just how they have failed as well as where they have been successful. Treatment modalities are rarely, if ever examined by anyone outside the paradigm or perspective: At least not until now. You will see how the "held notions" of past treatment providers have created the different perspectives and thereby the prescribed treatment of the addicted. As you read I'm sure that you will be able to understand each of the paradigms' possible benefits and even see how they might have created unintentional harm by their ignorance and inconsistencies.

At the end of this process we'll combine the successful and appropriate methods from each era/paradigm to establish a current more holistic approach to addressing the epidemic both for the addicted and by extensions his/her significant others.

A Foundation of Understanding

As all the truths about addiction are not yet known some of the points made in this chapter will be based on what is sometimes referred to in the legal system, under the constricts of evidentiary law as, "allowed by reason" or in layman's terms as "accepted knowledge." This is information that nearly everyone agrees on, like; smoking is bad for you, speeding is dangerous; addiction is painful. Simply speaking it is information that just seems obvious to everyone.

In examining the history of addiction I would like to suggest that anyone interested in some of the observations made in this book devote some more time and attention to an in-depth study of the various points made. Since this book's goal is to increase the understanding of the emotional aspects of addiction as a means of providing emotional relief, I will not provide much specific detail as this might distract from the book's primary purpose, which is again, treating the wounded.

Time Doesn't Heal all Wounds

One of the things I have found most interesting while working with addicts over the past 25 years is their amazing ability to justify their use. One of the ways they do this is by grasping onto the ideals of ancient societies that are believed to have used what are now illicit drugs. It seems as though their goal is to use this information to argue for a validation of use, the benefits of use or even for legalization of drugs like marijuana and other hallucinogens.

On the subject of legalization I ask you to consider a simple question: If cigarettes were illegal do you think that less people would smoke? Any honest person would admit that there would be less smoking, as some people will just not break the law. The age restrictions on cigarette purchases and restricted areas for smoking have already resulted in less use and thereby, less of a health problem. If the above premise is so, then how could the legalization of marijuana result in less of a problem? The only benefit would be to the addicts and criminals who refuse to accept their problems and to the legal system, which would then be absolved of the time and expense of prosecution. Let's not let them off the "hook" that easy.

While the legal system can be a great motivator for change and eventual abstinence, it is also partially responsible for our current failures. One could argue that a more strict legal system with greater penalties would be an even greater deterrent. Ask yourself this question: "Do you know anyone who was put in jail for a first offense of possession of marijuana?" I didn't say arrested, I said jailed or imprisoned, sentenced to time for their first substance offense? The held notion among users is that everybody "gets a pass" on the first charge. Is that a deterrent?

Further, much like cigarette smoking related diseases the legalization of marijuana would create an even greater burden on the medical and mental health systems, which are obviously already struggling with the problem. I will not address the issue of legalization any further as it is in my opinion a ridiculous idea spurred on by politicians seeking attention (i.e. political favor) and supported by a diseased and vulnerable segment of society blinded by their ambition to use. That segment being a small number of people who have smoked their way into denial, rationalization, immaturity, self-obsession, and self centeredness; who are most likely suffering from one of the most disastrous symptoms of marijuana dependency referred to as a-motivational syndrome.

You may also find it interesting to note that those ancient societies that used drugs such as the; Aztecs, Incas,

Mayans, and ancient Egyptians are all, just that, ancient. They failed to survive. While not yet an ancient society the American Indian also failed to maintain power over their own destinies and were it not for government intervention to separate them from society their fate may have been even more catastrophic.

While the connection between substance use and extinction may seem erroneous, these societies are still, for the most part, no longer with us. While many of these societies (American Indian excluded) used drugs for religious purposes, many of these practices became over exaggerated and even perverse leading to human sacrifice and the wasting of other resources vital to survival.

The Torah and the Bible both contain the book of Solomon in which the effect of excessive alcohol use is clearly described. The Book of Solomon may be one of the first credible written accounts of the negative effects of substance use on a society and maybe even on addiction itself.

Part II

Addiction Theory Over the Past 100 Years

This chapter examines the emotional and social perspectives of our society during the past one hundred years. It is this author's belief that only by examining these perspectives can we truly understand the current problems caused by addiction as well as the emotional struggles of the addicted and by extension, their loved ones. It will also give you a more thorough understanding of why you currently view addiction the way you do.

We will do this by examining how each of the models adopted by both governments and societies over the past one hundred years has affected both the substance user and their loved ones. We will also examine how some of these measures have actually been counterproductive resulting in today's misunderstanding of addiction and the wasting of valuable resources. While some of these models gained the majority of societal attention during their time and became mainstream approaches for a specific period, these models also occasionally overlapped. During this process you may also notice that sometimes different segments of society (governmental and religious) focused attention to the most provocative or culturally popular aspects of the problem in order to suit their individual ambitions and goals, usually at the expense of the addict and their family.

The Sinner

There are two major perspectives, which viewed substance use as a moral issue labeling the user with names like; degenerate, weak-willed, lush, bum, drunkard and even sinner. These models' names were self explanatory and fairly descriptive and were often referred to as part of the "Dry Moral Model" and the "Wet Moral Model" of addiction.

The <u>Dry Moral Model</u> saw drinking at any level as a sin of our lower nature. Many followers of this model believed that drinking was a weakness to evil forces and even an act against God. Alcohol was perceived of as a tool for the devil's bidding.

The <u>Wet Moral Model</u> relegated the sinfulness of drinking to those who drank too much or too often. Like the sin of Gluttony, those who over indulged faced the wrath of their own sins. Under this model it was not believed alcohol itself was inherently evil, only the over-use or overindulging. Both models believed that the user had and maintained a conscious choice in the matter of drink.

As mentioned above, the "Wet Moral Model" relegated the sin of drink to those who drank too much, drank at the wrong time, or who failed to stop before intoxication was reached. Both models believed that the user had a choice in the matter of drink and that those who became intoxicated, were committing sin; just like the adulterer or the thief, they acted and thereby chose to sin. Their suffering was of their own making. It was believed that the abuser would eventually stop after being motivated by the pains brought on by their own misdeeds. Under these models there was no understanding of the phenomena known as compulsion. Remember that during this era in our society there were no such things as kleptomaniacs, shop-a-holics, sex-addicts, no Obsessive Compulsive Disorders, or compulsive gamblers. There were no excuses or explanations for "bad" behavior beyond the individual. Individuals were held personally responsible for their shortcomings and society was not yet, to blame. Alcoholics and addicts were rarely treated or aided in their struggles as it was believed that by helping them the behavior was being condoned. Zero tolerance was the guiding force, which eventually lead to a constitutional amendment and prohibition. So strong were these beliefs that it changed our Constitution.

Dry Moral Model

If we take a closer look at the Dry Moral Model what it is suggesting is that alcohol use and/or by extension alcoholism was the result of a poor personal, family or societal value system. The alcoholic's parents, their church and their communities were believed to have failed in their duty to impart "real/true" values to the community and the individual. This theory epitomized the "It takes a village to raise a child" principle.

This era was unknowingly a very crucial period where the solution for the addiction problem may have serendipitously presented itself. Instead it was skewed by oversimplification of the problem and the religious fervor of the time. Common knowledge does suggest today that environmental conditions play a role in how people make choices. (Remember that at this time the genetic links to addiction were not yet imagined.) The village did indeed have an effect on the addict but unfortunately the reaction of the village/community was in hindsight counterproductive to the solution.

Despite their "good intentions" the creators of the Dry Moral Model's belief system and the holders of those beliefs are in a large part responsible for the overwhelming sense of shame many families of addiction (a disease) still experience today. Like the lepers of their day, these families were shunned while children were told not to relate with family members from those "types" of homes. This shaming and ostracizing only worsened the struggles of children from already troubled homes as they were now essentially cut off from the "positive" functioning of the healthier neighboring family systems. This paradox cultivated a climate that actually made the unfortunate children of alcoholic homes suffer more needlessly as now they themselves were also an unwanted segment of society. These children were innocent victims of the growing plague of addiction. It is quite possible that this type of ostracism led to more substance abuse by creating an outcast adolescent, poised to rebel against the society that shunned them and their family, thus creating more distance and only segmenting the society away from a unified community. The effect it had was to push these people further from the church that shamed them and away from a possible solution often found by recovering addicts today in the form of a Higher Power.

The Dry Morale Model also imparted an unfair and often inaccurate sense of responsibility on the family of the addict. While we now believe that family dysfunction can lead to high risk taking and using behaviors, which can eventually lead to addiction, the result cannot be exclusively correlated "in scientific terms" to the family's level of dysfunction. This erroneous correlation is simply eliminated by the mere fact/proof that not every abused child or child of a severely dysfunctional family becomes an addict or addicted. There is no provable direct cause and effect.

In this model the family was blamed because it was believed that alcohol use was a willful act of sin by the user. It was believed that the "sinner" should have been taught or have had modeled to them, better values by his or her family. It was "believed" by the proponents of this model that had these values been taught the user would have never indulged or overindulged in the first place. While practitioners of the Muslim faith may also agree that the use of alcohol is a sin against God, this model predominantly evolved from the belief systems of the Southern Christians of the time. Many of these practices and motivations for abstinence are still alive in the US and the world today.

The core belief here was/is that the devil often tempted people to commit sin and that addiction was the wrath of having given in to that temptation, as retribution for having sinned. It was believed that continued use allowed evil to grow stronger and that it eventually caused distress for the entire family; very representative of the adage "The sins of the father are cast out unto the son."

You should also consider that it was believed during the evolution of this model that alcohol affected everyone the same and that people with good morals and good values chose to not drink because of their love for God and by extension the love of their family and community.

It should be made very clear here that this author is not expressing any opinion about religious beliefs relating to alcohol consumption and that while the beliefs discussed may seem extreme, people and societies who subscribe to these beliefs reportedly suffer less of the per-capita ills of addiction by simply avoiding all use. They do however still get run over and killed by drunk drivers."

As has been previously suggested, these perspectives led to much of the momentum necessary to amend the US Constitution and establish Prohibition. Prohibition officially made what is now recognized as a disease, an illegal act. Those who suffered from this disease were considered criminals and not viewed as the ill people we believe them to be today.

Stop for a second and think about the amount of momentum needed to change the Constitution and you will still only be considering a small fraction of our society's fervor to rid itself of the scourges of alcoholism in the 1920's. This was a righteous fervor against a disease that tortures and kills more Americans per year than any war at any time in our history. A comparable amount of social momentum had not been seen or felt again in the United States until the attacks on 9-11.

As mentioned, Prohibition officially made the disease of addiction illegal to have. Think for a second. Can you imagine the United States of America outlawing a disease? Remember, an addict is an individual with a physiological/genetic/ metabolic/emotional disease who at that time was being judged because of a disease and called a sinner. The fallout of these beliefs in regards to negative stigmatism means that to this day you're still better off having a sexually transmitted disease then an addiction.

During this era it was believed that a religious conversion was the only way to get the user to change. The user had to come to believe that a relationship with God was more important than the brief relief of use. That by trusting in and waiting for God's grace, the user would come to feel a sense of wellness beyond that of the next drink or hit.

Remember, change is about behavior, healing is about a disease. This belief that addiction was a chosen misbehavior set the foundation for the criminality of addiction that still exists today. Unfortunately for the non-believer, no focus was given to the value of abstinence as a healing tool, in and of itself. A major difficulty with this perspective is that the intense level of shame experienced by the user often prevented them from presenting for the religious conversion (the cure) in the first place. Those persons, too filled with shame, just used more alcohol to overcome these feelings, these negative emotions and their negative self-concept. Today, many addicts still fail to seek treatment or ask for help due to this overwhelming sense of shame and remorse. That is the crime.

As in other models the user often fled their homes, jobs, and communities after their repeated attempts to hide their illness failed. This flight is believed to have created and fueled the large "Hobo" community of directionless train jumpers and anonymous street bums of the 20's and 30's. Addicts were forced to flee their home to prevent bringing shame on their families. In order to "save face" in the community families often created lies to explain where the family member had gone, often using stories of far away jobs, military service or even death.

Insights from this Model

- The belief that the use of alcohol was a sin and not a disease
- That alcohol effected everyone the same but that some people were more sin-full
- No one should drink and then the problem would not exist, like the views of nudity at the time, the mere presence of alcohol, tempted man beyond his personal strength.
- The only hope for change was through religious conversion. No was no real medical care or professional/clinical treatment
- Failure in this model resulted in major shame and diminished self respect leading to more use
- The alcoholic often gave in to the disease after religious conversion failed
- The alcoholic often fled their only support system, which could have been helpful to sustaining their recovery and abstinence efforts.

Morals with a Shot of Rationalization

While the Dry Moral Model may have been a little hard for the addict to swallow there was hope yet to come. This hope presented itself in what appeared at the time to be a new and revolutionary approach often referenced to in hindsight as the "Wet Moral Model." This model would revitalize the morality of drinking by allowing for the use of alcohol "in moderation." This was very exciting and optimistic news for a prohibition-ravaged society as well as to the struggling alcoholic who could not fathom life without alcohol. It is quite possible that this model evolved after the shock of prohibition settled in with the Northern Christians (Protestants and Catholics) who did not see drinking as a sign of weakness but instead frequently incorporated wine and "spirits" into religious services and positive celebratory occasions.

The hope for the alcoholic sprung from the suggestion that the use of alcohol could not only be continued but that the "drunkard" would actually be instructed on how to use successfully. This breakthrough was considered to be revolutionary at the time because the Wet Moral Model's "simple" aim was to teach the problem drinker how to consume alcohol appropriately. The addict would be taught the "rules" for drinking and this would somehow end their troubles with alcohol. (How about you, ever subscribe to this notion? Where did you think it evolved from? Now you know.)

While still morally centered it was in this model that society would take its first "non-religious" measures to address the problem (as Prohibition was indeed the result of religious fervor and pressure against consumption). In this model society sought an educational solution to the problem. There are some historical accountings that suggest agencies like the National

35

Institutes of Health sprung from these efforts as congress was lobbied to take action on the health problem of alcoholism in the shadow of prohibition's repeal.

Both members of society and the government as a whole would now begin to "teach" the alcoholic how to drink/use "properly." These supposed rules included; what age, how many, how often, what time, and what type or kind of alcohol to drink. This model suggested and believed that willpower was indeed the cure for willful misconduct. It was believed at the time that man had complete control over his physiology in regards to alcohol. Alcoholism was not yet recognized as a physical or health condition, but instead as a shortcoming of character, of failed insight and of poor decision making skills. Ideas related to obsession and compulsions were not widely understood.

As odd as it may seem to us now, some remnants of this philosophy still exist in many motor vehicle administrations around the country today where offenders are ordered to attend DWI classes and even the resolutely titled "Social Drinker Programs." Such titles only act to confuse the issue of addiction and to foster the often-preferred perspective that the drinker has only a current problem and not a chronic progressive emotional and physical disease.

One of the greatest shortcomings of this model is that it evolved from mainstream society's desire to explain the ills of drinking rather than treat them as the medical condition that it was then and still obviously is now. The model did not take into account the dangers of withdrawal, physical addiction or as mentioned above, compulsion. Because of the shortcomings in this model many people would die common alcoholic deaths from accidents, alcohol poisoning and complications of alcohol withdrawal. Many future death certificates would report heart attacks or heart stoppage as the primary cause of demise. (A heart attack is or can be an event of alcohol withdrawal; as the central nervous system depressant (alcohol) is removed the heart rate increases substantially, often leading to cardiac events.)

As might be expected "unacceptable" levels of use often continued as the alcoholics sought to treat their withdrawal symptoms. Unacceptable levels of use would be hidden or outright denied as it threatened societal perspectives on alcohol as well as this model's very core philosophies. Few citizens, or for that matter even those in the medical community, would dare to confront the issue of illness in a post prohibition era which often feared a return to the illegalization of alcohol, an increase in the organized crime and the mayhem that came with it. Even those persons in the medical profession who might proffer an alternate view during this era faced ridicule and scorn from their peers. One man who feared such scrutiny in a confused society wrote the chapter "The Doctor's Opinion" in the beginning of the book "Alcoholics Anonymous." Originally Dr Silkworth asked that his name not be included in the first edition for just that reason.

It could be argued that this model identified for us as a society and from a behavioral standpoint, how denial of the problem might prohibit confronting unacceptable behavior. The belief at the time was; if you lost control you had a problem and were then considered weak. Because of this, everyone including the user's family rationalized and justified the negative consequences of excessive use, eventually believing their own lies. Dysfunctional skills like rationalization, externalization, and blaming took flight. This model quite possibly retarded or postponed treatment advances and resulted in painful cycles of failure, remorse, suicide, broken hearts, abused children and devastated families.

By today's standards it is widely accepted that once a person loses control over their substance use they must abstain completely. In the Wet Moral Model the user just continued to beat their head against the proverbial wall of countless failures to regain control of their lives as they tried to "learn how to drink successfully."

I ask that you take a minute and try to think of any other disease where willpower is recommended as a form of treatment. Imagine if your doctor told you to use your willpower to control your blood sugar, to treat your diabetes; to stop letting your blood pressure rise so high; or even more preposterous to not smoke as much or to slow down your smoking to treat your lung cancer. While this comparison may seem ridiculous and extreme I remind you once again that alcoholism is a Chronic Disease in the same class as the aforementioned conditions. At a minimum, we should consider that a mental health issue like Bi-Polar or manic depression is a disease of the mind, but yet we still do not have the expectation that the sufferer can control his or her condition strictly by will. Our own struggle to group these problems together is evidence of our own still held misconceptions about alcoholism and addiction.

Wet Moral Model

- Alcoholics are simply not following the rules of drinking
- Social using becomes the goal
- Responsible drinking methods can be learned and even legislated (the drinking age)
- Society can rally to aid the alcoholic in non religious ways
- There were no agencies in place to provide this health education

38

- Willpower is all that is needed and believed to be a viable tool in fighting addiction
- The solution was a one pronged approach with a one model fits all solution
- Thousands suffer and die needlessly as the problem is ignored, hidden and even denied
- The wants/goals and denial of the many, ignores the plight of the few
- Model ignores physical withdrawal and physiological addiction and compulsion
- Since it suggests the person can keep using, many users do so and experience loss of control, dysfunction and death without the public's assistance or attention.

The Lush

Another model that we still seem to be under the influence of, first gained significant public attention in the old TV series "The Andy Griffith Show" and "Andy of Mayberry" in the character of Otis. This model, sometimes referred to as the "Impaired Model" viewed the alcoholic as suffering from a defect of birth which left the user unable to deny themselves when it came to the "choice" of, or control of, drinking. The belief here was that "drunks" (as they were frequently referred to during this time) could not change their destiny no matter what the intervention. While not the most promising of outlooks, the alcoholic was starting to be seen as less of a moral degenerate/sinner and more of a helpless person afflicted by a condition beyond his or her control. In truth, every treatment approach up to this point had failed miserably and this was the explanation brought forward to explain how the phenomena of alcoholism had eluded the religious, governmental and medical establishment's remedies. (Perhaps maybe even an expression of denial resulting from the inability of society to admit fault or failure.)

As portrayed in the TV series, the character of Otis was much loved by the community as is evidenced by the authority to lock himself in the Mayberry jail at night after an inevitable night of heavy drinking. This was not done for his or anyone else's safety, but instead to remove him from the public eye so that "good church going folks and their children" would not have to be confronted with his presence lying in the city streets on Sunday mornings. There was no believed fix for Otis's condition, just a remedy to the problem faced by society. There was now a growing and accepted truth that the Alcoholic was, is and would be an inevitable part of any social landscape, which allowed alcohol use among its members. The creators of the show are to be commended on their portrayal of Otis as an otherwise good person but none the less one with a real problem (Finally).

As has been suggested the societal view was one of helplessness. Thus, the alcoholic could no more be expected to take responsibility for removing himself from the eyes of children playing in the street then he could to avoid the consumption of alcohol. There were no treatment methods developed for the condition because it was believed to be a part of the users physical make up, a part of their core being, a genetic trait often traceable to a family history of like struggles. The alcoholic was now being recognized as a personality type with a family/genetic component not of their making. It was believed that no permanent change could be had and that no intervention would have any lasting effect.

There was also a societal assumption that once a certain age was reached without the presentation of a problem, then concern about future problems could be dismissed or eliminated. This was usually evidenced by; the "drinker's" being able to keep jobs, to look healthy, by being responsible citizen and by supporting their dependents/families. By believing the alcoholic was a type of "person" the rest of society could then consume alcohol with impunity, knowing that this unfortunate state could never happen to them as "they" had already proven to be productive member of society and not alcoholic lushes.

I am certain that many people reading this have heard or spoken the following sentence; "I don't have a problem, I pay my bills, I've never lost a job" and even, "I have a 700+ credit rating." All the prior are types and levels of denial suggesting that these evidences somehow make the individual immune to this disease.

Putting this model in perspective by today's standards of treatment we see that:

    a) The addict was believed to be a type of person who is suffering from a sort of genetic illness or disease

    b) A disease for which there was no cure

    c) Thus a disease, for which a cure would not need to be sought, as it was a permanent, untreatable condition

    d) These "users" weren't treated as second-class citizens; they were treated as the lowest class of citizens, a group of people with an inborn defect of will, they were treated much like the mentally retarded and mentally ill of that time:

    e) Users were people who where believed to have no ability to contribute anything positive to society and whose words and promises had to be ignored as wishful thinking.

Remember; "They just couldn't help it." The "diseased" individual would either be cast out by the family to spare the family embarrassment or would abscond to avoid bringing more shame to their families. Much like retardation at the time, this belief also created a stigma for the family whose genetic codes were now also suspect by friends and neighbors. Few parents of the time would eagerly seek to have their children marry into such problematic, "lower class" or even sub-par families.

The cumulative effect was the addict, now filled with shame and remorse from their sense of weakness as well as the shame projected on to them by society, would fall deeper into the cycle of intoxication in order to avoid feelings of worthlessness and inadequacy. The shame experienced by the user would eventually lead to either flight as a transient/hobo or as a suicide resulting from severe depression, which was seldom attributed directly to alcohol use.

Death by train was often considered to be a common accident of an alcoholic supposedly "falling asleep on the tracks" but in reality many of these "accidents" were the result of intentional self-harm and suicide. The death by train scenario would once again spare alcohol as the target, culprit or cause.

Avoid these misperceptions for yourself. Alcohol is a powerful drug, so powerful it can overcome almost any feeling as long as it is continuously being ingested. This vicious cycle of cause and cure often resulted in the alcoholic's flight from their hometowns to the larger cities. Except for the love of one addict to another the alcoholic would be met with even greater distain as they "invaded" new communities to which they were not members. The alcoholic was now a burden cast upon the big cities of America. Their commiseration with other "drunks" and their "flight response" to avoid conflict left them with even fewer options for change and still more justification of and even more need for their continued use of alcohol.

One of the greatest travesties of this model is that the substance problem was almost never identified until the latest stages of the disease, usually only after other major physical and psychological conditions had manifested. Because of societal ignorance early symptoms were not even considered because people hid their struggles in shame. This is the birth of the "Shame Based Disease Concept" which is believed by today's professionals to be the main reason people can't stop using and continue to relapse (more on this later).

Societies and the medical profession now know that any disease caught early in its formation has a better chance at a positive resolution. The further an alcoholic descends into the

43

depths of the disease the longer the recovery process must be. These "poor sots," victims of a disease were simply left to suffer the ravages of that disease. By all intents and purposes this once popular theory would only provide the user shelter and aid in their helpless struggle until they passed from either exposure to the elements, organ damage resulting from the effects of drinking, by suicide or even murder. It should also be mentioned that many alcoholics were blamed for crimes they did not commit because they were easy scapegoats/targets for law enforcement and for communities to which they did not belong.

This model suggests

- That they just can't help their addiction and that they are the victim of misfortune
- The condition is untreatable, people/society stopped looking for a solution
- It is inherited, the term genetic was not yet popularized
- Only identified in the very late stages of the illness
- The solution is to keep them away from children and society as whole by providing them shelter
- The prognosis was that they would probably die from alcohol use but if not they would certainly die with alcoholism
- The alcoholic accepts his destiny of shame, repeated binges, daily use and moves on to avoid family embarrassment.

Two Evolutions

During the next evolution in addiction treatment there were two models that evolved simultaneously. These two models are most often referred to as the 12-Step Model and the Old (or first true) Medical Model. The symbiotic relationship between these two models led to some major milestones in addressing substance dependency. For the first time emotional issues, personal perceptions and individual motivations for substance use would be investigated. Public health services, including the forerunner of the National Institute of Health would become better informed (through actual research) about the realities and dangers of alcohol abuse and dependency. These health agencies would begin a national public effort to educate the country on the ills of addiction, namely alcoholism. Sufferers of the disease would take responsibility for themselves, their behavior and their condition. These individuals would join together with the medical establishment in investigating and finding a resolution to the spreading plague of addiction.

For the first time the physiological and psychological aspects of the problem would be treated simultaneously. Educational methods would be used to try to aid the addicted and their loved ones in understanding the nature of their problem. Once safely detoxified by the medical community, the addicted would be taught how to treat their condition, repair the wreckage of their past, resolve their shame/guilt issues and maintain their abstinence. This union would give the addicted the necessary ingredients for change; hope and long-term support.

The "12 Step" Model
A Change in Lifestyle and Behavior

The 12 Step model evolved out of two earlier movements, one in the late 19th century called the Washingtonians and the other in the early 20th century called the Oxford Groups. The Washingtonians were focused on abstinence, strength in numbers and public education. The Oxford groups were a very well established "First Century Christianity" movement which contributed the idea that the Power found in God via spirituality and religion, could aid individuals to change and overcome their life struggles regardless of their socio-economic status. The Oxford Group movement was based on human compassion and public service. Oxford Group members hoped to unify the world using a set of practical spiritual principles, common values, personal principles and positive behavioral practices.

Early on in the evolution of the Oxford Groups they began working with suffering alcoholics from affluent families at the request of those families. The group was credited with an amazing record of lasting successes. Their simple belief in the ideals of; personal self appraisal, restitution for harms done, service to others, surrender to God and the seeking of God's Will would while minimalist, prove effective. They believed these spiritual principles could help anyone better develop and organize their life as they were convinced it was in keeping with what they referred to as "the natural order of things."

One of the cofounders of Alcoholics Anonymous, a man named William Griffith Wilson (an alcoholic) went on to write the book "Alcoholics Anonymous" as a synthesis of Oxford Group practices and personal successes. Mr. Wilson shares in the book of his experiences and successes while he tried to maintain his own abstinence via his work with other alcoholics. His first successful prospect was a doctor named Bob Smith. Once these two connected and found success the duo started reaching out to hospitals and asylums seeking alcoholics of their "type" to pass on their new practices and perspectives to. The message they carried was one of hope and fellowship. The power of proof was evidenced by their personal successes at staying sober "One Day at a Time." These two men maintained their Oxford Group connections for many years after their meeting.

As the numbers of recovering alcoholics grew and as they began to subgroup from the mainstream Oxford Group practices the "alcoholic squad" as they were referred to, was eventually encouraged to set out on their own with a primary focus of helping other alcoholics while improving their personal contact with a Higher Power. Thus, in 1935 the program of Alcoholics Anonymous was truly born with the meeting of these two men.

The Oxford groups remained supportive of their efforts and aided the fledgling program emotionally and spiritually in times of struggle. The 12 Steps as they are known today evolved during the writing of the book "Alcoholics Anonymous." The original 6 primary values used by Oxford Group alcoholics were expanded to the 12 steps as they are written today.

Other so named, "12-Step Movements" have obviously adopted the "12 Steps of Alcoholics Anonymous" as their guiding principles. Other 12 step programs now use the 12 steps to aid others in finding solutions to their addictions and a vast array of other problems related to powerlessness over troublesome compulsions. Movements, which have incorporated these practices, are now affectionately referred to as "12 Steps

47

Programs." These 12 principles (the steps) developed during this era are now put to work around the world facilitating recovery from many ills.

Unfortunately for the alcoholic still desiring to use alcohol and unlike the beliefs of the Wet Moral Model, this model advocated complete abstinence from alcohol. This was only accomplished with the promise and repeated reassurance that happiness and contentment could be found without alcohol if the practices of the 12-step program were followed closely. These men were literally living proof that alcoholics of their variety and severity could recover and be happy without alcohol.

Synchronistically, during the same time that the development of the 12 step program "Alcoholics Anonymous" was occurring, hospital programs in many of the larger cities around the country had been experimenting with what were euphemistically referred to as "drying out joints." These were usually special hospital units or wards dedicated to "safely" aiding the alcoholic through their detoxification process. For all intents and purposes they were psychiatric units. These drying-out joints began using various methods to ease the serious and fatal physical withdrawals experienced by alcoholics.

For the first time in the alcoholic experience the alcoholics were seen as suffering from a physical condition and not merely weak willed wrong doers, lushes or sinners. This reprieve gave many the needed motivation, understanding and release from shame necessary to begin the long road of personal recovery. For AA members, recovery is an ongoing process, one that is never completed. The disease is viewed as an illness like diabetes and heart disease, which are also chronic, progressive, irreversible and fatal if left untreated.

In the early years Alcoholics Anonymous focused their practices on the theories of a Doctor William Silkworth who proposed that the alcoholic suffered from a type of allergy to alcohol. This allergy of compulsion resulted in different responses to the chemical alcohol then those experienced by persons without the allergy. This allergy theory was an attempted explanation for the alcoholic's inability to moderate himself once the chemical was ingested. It was believed by Dr. Silkworth that a compulsion was experienced by the alcoholic that rendered his will power void. This is most easily understood when compared to a phenomena often referred to as the "potato chip principle," being that you can't have just one. This principle is an attempt to describe the compulsion of the alcoholic and addict for the second and successive drinks beyond "just" one or two.

The early members of AA believed that the compulsion experienced and created by the first drink was the same mental process used to rationalize and explain having another potato chip, peanut, etc, only much much stronger.

It should be noted that this level of compulsion grew as more and more was ingested, eventually overcoming all cravings for food as well as taking away the personal discipline to maintain daily life responsibilities. This failure was most often the very criteria used to label one an alcoholic. The AA literature speaks to this deficit as a "lack of power" (usually will power).

Much like hay fever or other allergies it was believed that some people just had the allergy and that nurture or life experience was not the cause. Like that of the hay fever sufferer who begins sneezing, the allergy theory proposed that if you had the allergy and reached the point of being overwhelmed by an agent (in this case alcohol) that the body could not recover its previous state until the overwhelming agent ran its course or was removed from the body.

Old timers in the AA program (people with long term recovery) often compared it to the cucumber and the pickle where; once a cucumber becomes a pickle it cannot go back to its original state because the organism had been altered by the agent, (i.e. pickled). Had it not been for the practices of the Oxford groups who focused on "well to do families," the nature instead of nurture aspect of this argument for a physiological cause may not have been pursued. During this time the influences of the previous moral models still played a major role in societal perspective. Ironically the greatest success ever attained over the ills of alcoholism, Alcoholics Anonymous, formed less than two years after the repeal of Prohibition.

The involvement of the 12 step members in this model resulted in one of the first efforts to treat the alcoholic both physically and emotionally. The AA program practice of "sponsorship" evolved from a collaboration and commitment between the medical treating establishment and the AA recovery community. Before a hospital would admit a destitute alcoholic for treatment they would require a commitment by a sober AA member to both visit the patient daily in order to provide emotional support and to accompany him upon his release from the hospital. This practice was instituted to decrease or at least retard the alcoholic's likelihood of returning to the bottle.

This model suggested:

- That there are many factors involved in causing and treating addiction
- That there are medical components of both substance use and detoxification
- That the alcoholic may actually have a type of allergy that causes them to lose control over their behavior and choices when exposed to the substance (ingested.)

- Some people have the allergy and some don't
- That the allergy causes a mental "OBSESSION" for the drug/chemical
- Once ingested the allergy created overwhelming compulsions for more
- That abstinence is the only true course of corrective action and that it takes regular interventions such as meeting with other alcoholics for reassurance and support to maintain that abstinence.
- That the success rate can be very high for those people who follow a prescribed path of clearing away the wreckage of their past and creating a new and rewarding life for themselves and their families.
- This model fits well into many of the other paradigms to create a more holistic approach to solving the problem.

The Old Medical Model

The first real version of the medical model was developed around the same time as the 12-Step model. This model believed that the cause of the malady resulted from the excessive use of the substance, in this case alcohol. It was believed in this model that the body eventually became overwhelmed by the chemical, reaching a state in which the human organism was permanently and irreversibly changed. The two major organs believed to be effected by alcohol use (at this time) were the liver and the brain.

The medical establishment at the time determined through experience working with suffering alcoholics that their bodies had become damaged by the use of the alcohol. Once the organ systems of the body were damaged the choice in drink was lost as the body could no longer tolerate or metabolize the alcohol properly. Medical professionals theorized that the body's failure to metabolize the alcohol (via the liver) resulted in abnormally high blood alcohol content for extended periods, which then altered and damaged the brain's functioning. When the alcohol was then removed (by attempts to abstain) the body went into a form of shock now known to most of us as withdrawal or abstinence syndrome. This was proved after the resulting withdrawal or shock was quickly reversed by the administration of more alcohol or another like substance (a drug from the same class.) Thus the first provable criteria for chemical dependence was established known now as; "withdrawal-syndrome."

During this time it became increasing apparent that alcohol was "not good for the body," and that drinking alcohol just once, (in extremely large doses) could cause death.

Unfortunately the medical profession at the time was not in concert with the psychological profession so emotional support and counseling was not yet readily available. It should also be mentioned that the majority of indigent alcoholics could not afford psychological or psychiatric help.

While doctors and nurses provided emotional support, their focus remained on the physical (clinical) aspect of the illness. Addiction was not yet being recognized by the medical profession as a physiological and psychological illness but instead only as a medical condition, a cause and effect syndrome. Methods were focused on convincing the addict through fear, to stop using or face certain and inevitable death. "If you continue to drink you will die." This is effective unless the person wants to die or is unable to see a road to recovery.

During this time the disease of addiction was only being identified in the later stages. A clear criteria for identifying problematic use had not yet been considered. The idea of a harmful pattern of use was not yet identified or established because members of our society still sought to shamefully hide their use until the problem was undeniable or very obvious and it was then, often too late to intervene.

The physical discomfort created by the withdrawal of the late stages of the disease often found the addict returning to the vicious cycle of use in order to gain some type of relief. I once met a man named Ray who stated that during the 1930's and 1940's he had been repeatedly admitted to what were then referred to as "drying out joints" (mentioned earlier). These were the alcohol treatment centers of the day. He told me that once after he had completed a so-called hospital "drying out" program and was being discharged, the staff waved goodbye to him and said, "See you next time Ray." The medical community had accepted that the cycle would continue. A treatment or intervention process to stop the cycle was not yet suggested or practiced: At least not until the formation of Alcoholics Anonymous.

The most important development that evolved from this model

- Excessive drinking caused the problem or condition
- Once the body was damaged by alcohol, control over choice in drink was lost
- People were beginning to view alcohol from a clinical perspective, removing the moral implications of the problem (a vital change)
- The physiological treatment mechanisms of addiction were finally being investigated
- The solution might require long term interventions
- The medical profession began to focus and refine what their role would be in the process
- Without psychological intervention many alcoholics would just resolve to using for the rest of their lives

A BIG MERGER

Thus we arrive at an important point in history when the two models; the 12 Step Model and Medical Model (emotional and medical) merge in an effort to create a more holistic model of treatment. This was the alignment of two forces that would begin treating the alcohol addiction problem from multiple fronts; the spiritual, the emotional and the physical. This merger was the first step towards the eventual evolution of our current treatment approaches. This merger was just the beginning of our exploration towards a humanistic and holistic solution.

These two communities of care would then inspire other concerned persons, interested parties, medical professional and mental health practitioners to create an even more integrated approach to treatment. This merger would give birth to and enable specific areas of expertise to be created and evolve regardless of the shortcomings of other weaker aspects of any particular paradigm. The baby would no longer be thrown out with the proverbial bath water and the all or nothing practices of previous models would be "tempered" and expanded upon.

The following chapters discuss these areas of focus. They do not suggest that the other approaches that evolved at the same time are not valid; they simply focus on different causes and solutions from different perspectives. As you read you will certainly see how aspects of these theoretical paradigms and their insights have led us to our current and possibly even our future understanding of this complicated issue.

Psychodynamic Model

The Psychodynamic Model began to gather serious momentum during the late 70's and early 80's as some of the benefits of Freudian counseling techniques gained credibility. This specific model of psychotherapy and counseling suggested that in its most fundamental state addiction was merely one of the "Personality Types" which naturally evolved due to specific environmental influences. It suggested that people could develop a type of personality disorder, which resulted in their returning to a specific behavior (drinking in this case) for either escape or relief. The "Addictive Personality" as it was labeled, was reported to have certain factors or traits, which spanned the multitude of possible addictions. In the early 1980's the National Academy of Sciences suggested that several key elements had been identified to establish an outline for what they called the Addictive Personality.

These elements included but are not specifically limited to the following:

- Impulsive behavior
- Difficulty in delaying gratification
- Some antisocial personality traits (we know today this was apathy)
- A disposition toward sensation seeking
- A high value on nonconformity combined with a weak commitment to the goals or achievements usually valued by a society
- A sense of social alienation and a general tolerance for deviance
- A sense of heightened stress and catastrophizing

The psychodynamic model believed that unsuccessful developmental transitions and traumatic events left some individuals more susceptible to developing the Addictive Personality type, suggesting that difficulties during these transition periods reflected higher incidences of addiction manifestation. More generally speaking (in regards to the Psychodynamic Model) it was unanimously agreed that the alcoholic and drug addict were suffering from some underlying unresolved psychological conflict. Addiction was believed to only be a symptom of the "real" problem. It was believed that if the underlying conflict or "real problem" could be resolved, the addictive personality behaviors would then cease.

In this model the addiction problem would most likely be addressed in psychotherapy, also known and referred to as long-term counseling and psychoanalysis. While the term counseling is often used in regards to psychotherapy, not all counseling techniques use psychotherapy techniques to address core issues. Psychotherapy is often seen as a longer process to examine the client's transitional stages and adjustments to the life cycle to uncover the "misstep" experienced during an individual's development. This is a technique that requires a vast understanding of both the developmental processes as well as the awareness of the various factors that contribute to this misstep or failure to progress through a developmental stage successfully.

Unfortunately by today's standards most people can neither afford the investment required to attain this level of care nor are they willing to give the process the level of openness, motivation and time necessary to attain these insights and healing. Until these processes are completed there is usually little change in "Behavior," (ie; drinking pattern.) It has only recently become clear to the counseling professions that medicating addicts is only a temporary solution used to give the therapeutic or counseling process a chance to acquire necessary insights for the client to work though these various stages.

There are several major limitations to an approach that only operates from the Psychodynamic perspective. The first relates to the personal insights and skills of the therapist or counselor. In order for a therapist to aid an addict successfully they must understand the machinations of the addict mind and thus have experience with the framework of defense mechanisms from which an alcoholic or addict operates. The therapist's knowledge of normal human behavior and human development is only minimally helpful at best.

Therapists working to uncover these deep seated core issues of shame and guilt must be able to foresee the painful effects of this new awareness and balance it with the addicts unique ability to self deceive. Unwatched and unrecognized the addict will eventually become adverse to the techniques being used because they are leaving their sessions without closure on specific subjects with high relapse potential. The addict mind tends to dwell on negativity, often leading to states of hopelessness and suicidal ideation. When this occurs in the mind of the addicted the best hoped for outcome for the addict becomes a return to use as their negativity often evolves into suicide ideations.

The process of psychoanalysis requires a level of trust and willingness only found in addicts in serious crisis. The therapist must be able to strongly confront inconsistencies in the user's report and then provide alternative perspectives, which are more functional ways of viewing the problem. Many therapists believe that this confrontation goes against they're understanding of the therapeutic process itself. In these cases the therapist has to ethically consider the limitations of their own bias. An installation of HOPE is indispensable but not often a part of the psychoanalytic practice. The psychoanalytic practitioner most often operates from an approach built around "free association," where the client is left to make most of the decisions about what topics are discussed and processed. The therapist must be able to highlight issues of self-deception (discussed later.) Further, since the reasons and motivations for using a substance often shift in meaning for the addict the original impetus for using may become moot and the use may become more behavioral in nature. In this model the initial cause for use is the total focus of the presumed solution and not the possible and likely changes of motive for the patient's current use. In most models "substance use" is seen as the primary problem and a disease with its own associated symptoms. This model often suggests that addiction is merely a symptom of a psychological problem. (This dilemma is addressed later in the Bio-Psycho-Social model)

Once again, this model suggests that addiction is emotional in nature. It does not specifically provide for measures to confront the obvious physical addiction, behavioral conditioning and withdrawal often associated with relapse. Once physically addicted the addict or alcoholic has changed their body chemistry in regards to how a substance like alcohol is metabolized and processed. Controlled use, often the goal in this model usually fails miserably. When controlled use is attempted the shift in "motivation to use" from the initiating transitional failures takes hold and is rekindled as if the addict never stopped. The new motivations for use that developed during addictive use and the prior conditioned attachment of the reward cycle of use, are now the cause of the problem and not the initial pathology that lead to the addictive use in the first place.

A simple example would be the 35-year-old female cocaine addict who has been detoxed and who has since, with the help of counseling, healed from her abusive past. She has become so used to the dramatic ups and downs that she now dislikes her current "flat" emotional state. She may also dislike the physical changes she is now experiencing such as weight gain. Many female cocaine addicts report that because they were "thinner" while using their perception is that they were more attractive when using. This "newly" developed motivation may be content for the counseling session but will rarely be resolved easily because it is further complicated by other "rewards" of use.

A second example might be that in a male addict, say a 35-year-old man who now enters recovery but finds himself unable to comfortably talk to women sober as it was previously only accomplished while intoxicated. He becomes unable to address this loneliness he now feels. He now finds himself intimidated to approach women while sober. One drink to "loosen up" returns him to his physical compulsion to use. This social discomfort and awkwardness needs to be addressed in counseling. Too often important issues like this become lost to the seriousness of the addiction itself. This shift in motivation would suggest that his current use has little to do with his initial motivations to begin use. That's what I mean by complicated.

The above two examples are what I refer to when I say that new motivations for use present themselves during the addictive process. Simply addressing the initial cause of use becomes almost irrelevant. It is true that these other issues can be counseled but that is not necessarily a part of this model.

This model's highlights
- Addiction is caused by an underlying psychological conflict resulting from an unsuccessful transition through a life or developmental stage
- Addiction is only a symptom of a personality problem

- Psychotherapy in needed to resolve that personality problem
- The process requires a therapist also experienced in addiction
- The shortcoming of the model is that new reasons and motivations for use evolve over the course of the addiction onset
- Lifetime abstinence is not the focus,
- Abstinence is only required during the change or resolution period

Dysfunctional Family Model

The supporters of the Dysfunctional Family Model believe that much like in the Psychodynamic Model, negative environmental issues nurture the development of an addictive personality and addictive behaviors. This model suggests even more specifically that the addictive personality is produced by family environmental factors rather than social environmental factors.

This model purports that family dysfunction and the human reactions related to that dysfunction, lead to the development of a "survival based personality type." They believe this to be an extremely common occurrence in the Dysfunctional Family, and it is aptly termed the "Addictive Personality." Once again this is a personality role that is formed as a method to deal with or cope with, the stressors brought on by high levels of family dysfunction, of which abuse is an extreme example.

Proponents of this paradigm believe that there is a very predictable pathology, which determines the level of dysfunction responsible for the development of and nurturing of this role. It should be noted that all families have some level of dysfunction and that when identifying a family as dysfunctional this model is referring to those with abnormally high levels of dysfunction in certain key areas. These areas include; externalization, rationalization, justification, blaming, avoidance, denial, projection, abuse of all types, extreme self-centeredness, and parental personality disorders. Parental or guardian addiction is believed to just carry dysfunction forward from the previous generation.

As mentioned above some types of dysfunction are present in all families. Some of the more problematic areas include; modeling of the addictive personality, codependency in a primary caregiver, lack of emotional support when coping with personal struggles, and the failure to pass on positive functioning tools for the resolution of personal problems and personal stressors. Also problematic are issues around family denial of problems/avoidance, physical health, violence, and as mentioned emotional/physical/sexual abuse. In this model all of the aforementioned types of dysfunction are believed to contribute to the development of the addictive personality.

Treatment providers who work in this paradigm believe that the addict role can be addressed by helping the family increase their level of positive functioning. The individual's maladaptive behaviors including substance use must also be addressed individually in treatment. This model proposes that the family engage in family therapy to address the dysfunctional system as a whole. It would be considered by this author to be almost unethical not to address family function problems in all models, once identified. In most cases this type of family therapy involves the identification and labeling of dysfunctional patterns and then aiding the family in ceasing those dysfunctional patterns. Once that is done the family is then educated and supported while they practice and incorporate more positive ways of functioning.

Anyone who has a family can attest that this process sounds much simpler then it is. Unfortunately once dysfunctional patterns are established within a family the family often becomes segmented and they have difficulty unifying for the therapeutic process to begin and take place. Too often members of highly dysfunctional families learn how to get their needs met outside of the family of origin and are resistant to investing time and energy into what is perceived as a lost cause.

Treatment becomes increasingly more difficult if the addictive personality has already embarked on a pattern of

63

substance use, abuse and dependency. One of the major stumbling blocks to overcoming these obstacles is the existence of DEEP-seated resentment. Dysfunctional families often adapt the habit of using resentment to make other family members pay for, or suffer for, their prior misdeeds and misbehaviors. It is a common practice to withhold affection as a penalty for unacceptable behaviors. Members of these families who seek out treatment also learn and realize that separating themselves from their families is a method of protecting themselves from further emotional injury, thus they are resistant to participate.

These dynamics make uniting the family for treatment difficult at best. More often than not the level of protest experienced within the family to confronting their problems and changing their behaviors wins out: The family chooses to avoid facing the issue often choosing to blame the addict or an individual family member instead of the whole system.

For the proceeding reasons this model does not experience a high level of success. It is important to note that regardless of how addiction starts, once started other motivations for use are developed. An addict who has surrounded themselves with a group of other substance abusers is not likely to give up their using friends (their new dysfunctional family) for one that has already failed them. While some progress might be made, the failure of the user to sever ties with other users often results in an eventual relapse. Physical addiction is a medical fact. During withdrawal the user's body develops a craving and compulsion for the drug. A happy, positively functioning family will not be enough to treat the medical aspects of an addiction. Changing the family only decreases the development of more addictive personalities and reduces future stressors, it does not change the emotions or the behaviors now present in the addict.

Over my more than 25 years of working with addicted families it has become blatantly apparent that the users often develop more reverence for a relationship with the drug then with what seems like only a possible successful relationship with their family of origin. The addict often views the drug as the thing that saved their life after what their families "did" to them. The addict will even sometimes verbally state their plan to keep using until the family system changes. This is obviously irrational.

As a reader of this book I would like you to be sure of one very important fact. Addict or not, substance use on any level, retards the types of emotional growth sought in a therapeutic process. If anyone hopes to heal more quickly, from an emotional struggle of any kind, they should avoid all "mood altering" substances.

This model suggests the following
- The cause of addiction is a result of family emotional dysfunction, and a pathological family system which does not meet its members' needs
- The addict is a role that develops within a dysfunctional family and is a natural occurrence within the dysfunctional family system
- The goal of treatment is to reduce the dysfunction in the family and thereby eliminate the stressors that require substance use in the first place
- The method is rarely successful at uniting the family for treatment purposes
- This paradigm only focuses on the original motivations for use and not the motivations that develop after the use begins

The Love Model

An old Beatles song suggested: "All you need is love." Well, if you believe that then this model will make a lot of sense to you. Supporters of this paradigm believe that the addict develops a pattern of using to cope with a deficit of caring, nurturing and loving support. Much like the aforementioned "Family Dysfunction Model," this model suggests that nurturing and loving have a role in the development of a healthy individual (psyche) and that insufficient love causes problems like addiction.

The distinction between the Love Model and Family Dysfunction Model is that the nurturing in this model need not come from any specific source (the family) and that even if a family system does not provide the love needed, that other environmental factors such as religious and social interactions can compensate for a dys-functioning family. The belief in the Love Model is that people who have gleamed the benefits of positive nurturing develop self-concepts that can overcome the stressors that often lead to addiction and that people who have the necessary amounts of love in their lives are less susceptible to influences like peer pressure.

While this model is an effective addiction prevention strategy the maladaptive behavior patterns of the established addict can and will be used by the addict to exploit efforts to help them change making this model fall far short of its intended goal. Because of the desperation most addicted persons experience they are often blinded to issues of right and wrong and are instead clouded by issues of entitlement, victimization selfishness and self-preservation.

An addict, once "in his cups" will merely become gluttonous on the influx of attention, sympathy and resources provided to them, only exploiting the love and support to continue and prolong their using. While recovery programs preach living one day at a time the using addict has perfected this philosophy in reverse leaving the work of building a real life to another day. The "I'll get clean tomorrow" syndrome can be easily put into perspective by remembering the cigarette smoker who rambles on about how he needs to quit. Why isn't he quitting today if he truly believes he needs to quit?

WARNING: If you learn nothing else from this book, believe it when I tell you, you cannot love them clean and sober. While AA and NA may purport to "love them till they can love themselves" this only references the giving of support, hope and encouragement for the person who is personally committed to abstinence. The emptiness of addiction is a sort of emotional black hole void of a bottom until the "user" stops using both drugs and people. Detoxification, education, and rigid boundaries must precede the caring and compassion that will only be helpful once the addict commits to, and makes fundamental changes.

The majority of Drug and Alcohol Prevention strategies in place in the US today have evolved from the same beliefs held within this paradigm but they are "Prevention Strategies" and not treatment strategies. Drug prevention strategies seek to provide the children of addicted/dysfunctional parents the loving resources they need to overcome the obstacles experienced due to the dearth of function, love and attention. .

This model suggests addictive behavior results from issues related to poor/low self-esteem, and diminished self worth due to inadequate caring and even neglect. Deficits of the aforementioned levels of self worth and self respect predispose a child to the acceptance of initial dangerous risk taking behaviors, like substance experimentation. It is this author's experience

68

that "self-efficacy" is the best inoculation against peer pressure but that it does little for the currently addicted other than to make them better at attaining their drug of choice. Children who have healthy self-efficacy levels don't make poor decisions based on wanting or needing to feel accepted and worthy. Self-efficacy issues are usually related to missed opportunities like success in sports that would or could develop "personal resilience," (another natural inoculation against peer pressure). However, it is in reality only the early stages of substance experimentation that are avoided with healthy self-esteem and self-worth. Once the line of experimentation has been crossed the complicated dynamics of behavioral conditioning, rewards both personal and social, make complete avoidance rare and addiction more likely.

This model focuses on the following:

- Addiction occurs because people don't love themselves enough to take care of themselves and avoid dangerous risk taking behavior like using
- This lack of care results from not being adequately cared for or from actual abuse
- Excessive use is the result of poor self concept and low self-esteem
- The goal is to get the person nurtured and loved, have them enter into healthy relationships and support groups to learn their value (service work)
- Doesn't account for physiological addiction issues or secondary reasons for use, only the initial cause
- Creates an unrealistic sense of guilt in care givers
- The blaming of others for their lack of nurturing can result in a lack of personal responsibility for their

condition, resulting in justified use and more negative behaviors

Behavioral Model

As the name implies this model is based on the larger paradigm of the Behavioral Learning Model. Popularized and often sited to explain this model are the experiments of Ivan Petrovich Pavlov (1849-1936.) In his experiment Pavlov used a dog as the main test subject of his research. Pavlov was awarded the once valued Nobel Prize for his research on this subject. Quite simply; Pavlov rang a bell then fed the dog. He did this over and over again. Early on in his experiment he noticed that the dog would only salivate when the food was presented. As the research progressed he started noticing that the dog began to salivate before the food was presented, at the stimulus of the ringing bell. He thus discovered the concept and coined the phrase of "behavioral conditioning," now widely accepted as one of the major models for human learning and by extension human behavior.

A more scientific view might look like this: Pavlov noticed that the dog (the test subject) began to salivate when the stimulus was applied (the bell being rung) and before the reward (the food) was actually presented. As mentioned above he termed this state "Behavioral Conditioning." The dog was conditioned to believe that the bell meant that food was going to follow. Thus a reward would be attained or experienced. A stimulus (the bell) brings on a predictable response to the conditioning (salivation) after repeated exposure, hence a "conditioned response." He documented that the behavior would even continue without the presentation of the food. He continued this process until the salivation stopped; he termed this phase of unlearning, "Extinction."

Pavlov would later expand this research by including the terms "positive and negative conditioning." Positive

71

conditioning would bring on a behavior and negative conditioning would stop or extinguish a behavior. Anyone who has ever had a child or even a pet is quite familiar with these processes of reward and consequence. (Hopefully)

When this model is applied to addiction theory it quite simply suggests that addiction is the result of either learned behaviors (watching others) or conditioning through the repeated rewarding of a behavior; or as described above, conditioned response. If children grow up watching people using a chemical to cope with life stressors, life celebrations and other life situations, it is believed that they will model these behaviors later in life. The belief is that if a child sees dad come home from work each day and reward himself with a nice cold beer that these behaviors will not only be modeled later in life but that they will often be interpreted as a sign of success and maturity. Even without the actual practicing of the behavior (doing it) it can be intuited by observation alone that it is a reward for working hard or even a rite of passage into adulthood itself. It is believed that many male and female roles are learned behaviors adapted through modeling by parents. In life and in this model, substance use and addictive use patterns are only one of the practices often modeled and learned through observation.

The modeling of these use patterns sets the stage in such a way that it almost predisposes the individual to later practice these behaviors as well. Once the actual use begins the behavior is reinforced much more quickly because of the chemical reward. It should be noted that some geneticists argue that some behaviors are instinctual and not learned at all. Practitioners who work in this model build their treatment approaches around reward and consequence. One of the core practices in treatment programs based on this model is the old adage; "We can't think our way into right living, we have to live our way into right thinking," as time is required to un-condition the addiction. Because this is such an important concept and a major aspect of human learning the process of behavioral conditioning will be discussed in more detail in later chapters.

Before we depart from the subject for now; I think it is important that I give you one more consideration on this model. Over the past 20 years or so we have often heard experts claim that cigarette smoking is harder to quit then heroin. Yes and no. The suggestion here is that because of the frequency of reinforcement, the behavior and the following reward, the "behavioral addiction" if you will, is greater for the smoker than the heroin user. The heroin/opiate user might administer the drug 20 times in a day but the cigarette smoker administers the chemical as many as 20 times per cigarette, times 20 cigarettes per day. As an aside it is also true that the faster a reward is delivered following a behavior the more reinforced it is. By example, rewarding or disciplining a dog 10 minutes after an event would be useless. The quicker the condition is applied the stronger the "emotional connection" (addiction).

Insights from this model

- Children learn behaviors from their primary caregiver through modeling
- The benefits of use can be inferred without ever having actually used the chemical
- If modeling is followed by actual practice the behavior becomes even more emotionally valued
- That it takes time to extinguish a behavior and that there must be a negative consequence or negative condition to devalue the reward initially sought and experienced.

New Medical Model/ Chronic Disease Model

To put it simply the New Medical Model/Chronic Disease model is the current evolution of the medical profession's research and findings in regards to addiction. While the model is in a constant state of metamorphosis its foundation remains the same. (Once again I remind the reader that this book is not a technical review of the medical aspects of addiction. Our goal is to understand the emotions and thought process of the addict. The American Medical Association (AMA), The National Institute on Drug Addiction (NIDA) and The American Society of Addiction Medicine (ASAM) are great resources for those interested in finding and examining addiction from a more medical health perspective.)

In the Chronic Disease model it is believed that two major factors are at play in regards to how and why addiction presents. Chronic addiction is seen as the result of either predisposition or as the result of pathological organ changes that occur due to excessive use over an extended period of time. Once the addictive state is achieved the body cannot reverse the condition and the user is considered for all intents and purposes, to have now "contracted" the disease of addiction. In the recovery communities the word "disease" is often broken down as follows by saying; the body is at Dis---Ease with itself, as in "not" at "ease" with itself. This play on words is a brilliant insight into the emotional status of the addict as well as on how they are almost never comfortable unless they are using.

This model uses the medical establishment's terms and condition to explain addiction. It sees a chronic disease as a morbid process that has very characteristic symptoms. As with many diseases the etiology or cause is not always known.

74

Regardless of causation most diseases have a determinable prognosis (meaning what will happen if the progression is allowed to continue.)

A morbid process is something that shortens a person's life span and causes premature death. Not everyone who has cancer dies from cancer. They can still have other issues that end their lives from getting hit by a car, to addiction and even suicide but they still have it when they die. In this model it is believed that since their body has changed as a result of use the addict will take their dis-ease to their death. They might not die from it but they will die with it.

As mentioned above, this model suggests there is a very predictable course of symptoms and events that will occur as a result of the illness, hence the term pathology. This pathology can be easily measured and defined. The term "Chronic" is borrowed from the medical perspective. A condition is usually seen as either Chronic or Acute. Acute conditions have a sudden onset and exist for a limited amount of time. Persons with acute conditions either get cured of the problem or die from it in a short period. The individual usually has no role in acquiring the condition and they are usually curable. Appendicitis is a great example of an acute illness or disease state. It happens quickly, you go to the hospital to get if fixed (removed) or you die from it in a short time. Once it's fixed you no longer have a problem with it and it's considered resolved or cured.

Chronic conditions are almost the opposite of acute conditions. The chronic condition starts slowly and builds over time. Symptoms of these conditions can come and go over time but increase in their presentation and frequency. While the symptoms may come and go there is a constant threat of death or disability. People with chronic illnesses usually delay seeking treatment due to the mild presentation of some of the primary symptoms and as with most chronic diseases the patient often resists following the advice of their doctor once the disease is identified. Just ask any Diabetic who eats sugar or any Heart Disease patient who eats steak and excessive sodium (a type of denial, more later).

Chronic diseases are seen as "Primary" illnesses that are; "Progressive," "Fatal" and even easily diagnosed which is referred to in this model as "Simple." In this model there are easily identifiable stages, usually referred to in a simple format of early, middle, and late. This model identifies/views the "Early Stage" of addiction by; relief use, blackouts, getting a DUI/DWI and the beginning of Loss of Control (choice over how much is used and when.)

The Middle Stage is represented by increasing life difficulty as the result of use, including but not limited too; family problems, school problems, employment problems and more serious legal problems like violations of probation and domestic violence.

The "Later Stage" is mostly used to identify the results of serious physical deterioration. This includes almost any type of organ damage; liver, pancreas, brain damage etc....

Primary Symptoms

In the Chronic Disease Model there are two types of symptoms that present. Primary Symptoms often considered "Covert" in nature (not visible) and Secondary Symptoms seen as "Overt" in nature (obvious.) These symptoms have a tendency to wax and wane in their presentation often suggesting to the user that they might not have their malady after all. This cessation of symptomology is a great motivator for the addict desiring to use and it provides a rationalization for a return to use, what might be called the "I'm all better now" syndrome.

The Primary (Covert) Symptoms are as follows: The first is easily diagnosable; that of Tolerance. Most people in our society have heard this phrase used in regards to addiction. Most people see this as the "ability" to use more or "handle" more of something. People who can drink someone else under the proverbial table have a "higher tolerance." Tragically this is seen as an advantage in certain social circles and not as the covert presentation of a symptom of a disease. Having tolerance does not necessarily mean that the person is an addict; much like having a cough does not mean that a person has lung cancer or emphysema. Regardless of the severity it is a symptom of the disease.

Tolerance exists in two types. The first type has already been identified as the "ability" or the "need" to drink more alcohol to get the desired effect, often referred to as Metabolic Tolerance. The second type is often referred to as Behavioral Tolerance. This is seen as a diminishment in the appearance of the normal effects of use. This means the individual does not look drunk or high and that they function somewhat normally considering their level of intoxication. What is occurring here is the user's brain and body have adapted to the chemical and have learned how to compensate for the actual poisoning done by the chemical. This is the person whose eyes no longer get red, they no longer stagger when walking and they can function fairly "normally" while under the influence. This is only one explanation of how some alcoholics can drive their vehicles with blood alcohol levels that should be inducing coma (.30 or higher.)

The next symptom on the checklist is sometimes referred to as Cellular or Tissue Adaptation. This must occur in order for the Behavioral Tolerance to present. This is when the body moves towards incorporating the amount of a substance used

77

into the body's daily operations and functions. Once this occurs the state of withdrawal is experienced much more severely and it creates the condition referred to as "Chemical Dependency" (more later.) This is where more serious bouts of "loss of control" present as well. The addict no longer controls their substance use; it now controls them. They lose choice over when they want to use, where they want to use, how much they plan on using and for how long.

This Primary and Covert symptoms of addiction in the Chronic Disease Model, are known by the mainstream of mental health professionals, as Physical Dependence. Because of the frequent level of use by the addict the body now believes that the substance is a necessary nutrient and is required to maintain the current homeostasis. The body has, in essence created a false homeostasis. When the chemical is taken out of the body (via lack of administration of the chemical) the dependent experiences a type of shock called withdrawal. This is identifiable by actual physical reactions like changes in heart rate, sweating, blood pressure, shaking etc... By re-administering the same or a like chemical substance and seeing if the symptoms subside we can easily diagnose a physical dependence state. This cessation of symptoms is usually quite fast.

Once an addict gets to this stage the proverbial horse is out of the barn. When the user begins treating their withdrawal by using more, the benefits of using the drug creates an emotional/mental illness. This is when the user will often need inpatient and/or medical treatment and supervision to abstain as they have sold themselves on the idea that the drug is a necessary part of their feeling OK with the world. These now held fallacies make the chemical dependent very resistant to abstinence. They will guard their substance use with great passion, much like the starving man clings to his last piece of bread.

The last of the Primary Symptoms is very simply titled "Pathological Organ Change." This process is almost never diagnosable to medical testing in its early stages due to its subtle nature. These changes are slow and build over time (Chronic) usually only being found in the later stages of their progression, often when it's too late to reverse or slow the organ change/damage down. They include but are not limited to liver impairment and disease, nutritional deficiencies, Central Nervous System deterioration, lowered resistance to infection, pancreatitis and real brain damage (damage to the neural networks in the brain.)

Secondary Symptoms

The placement of the following symptoms as secondary is a little confusing because they are usually noticed first. Briefly put they are secondary in seriousness relating to the physical body. While still troublesome they are seen as psycho-social causes or conditions and hence secondary in a Medical model. This does not mean that they are not very serious; quite to the contrary; they can induce death to both the user and to others around them, not to mention the threat of long-term incarceration. Remember, these are "Overt" symptoms and should raise serious flags about addiction states in loved ones.

The first of the secondary symptoms we'll examine more closely is generalized to "Legal Problems." These legal problems run the gambit but the two most prevalent are DWI (driving while intoxicated) and drug possession. The others include things like burglary, theft, robbery, trespassing, domestic violence, murder, etc... Unfortunately many of these symptoms are gauged in their seriousness by how hard they are to resolve

79

within the legal system. These symptoms are glaring warning signs of a major loss of control looming in the user's future.

The next "Secondary Symptom" is referred to as "Interpersonal problems." Interpersonal problems are identified as problems relating to significant figures in one's life. They include spousal discord, problems relating to parenting children, to struggles getting along with friends and co-workers. While some of these relational problems may result in legal complications, in this model legal problems are simply seen as a progression of interpersonal problems. These can include arguments over meeting your responsibilities to gross failures like being late for important events or forgetting to pick your children up from school or baseball practice. This is the symptom that gives birth to and is most likely the seat of family dysfunction in the realm of addiction. This is where the true hurt takes place for those people around the addict who are only seeking to understand the believed "irrational behaviors." These problems are not cognitive issues but instead they are early symptoms of the disease. In this model these struggles are seen as a disease state and not an emotional reaction or an issue of responsibility, priority or propriety.

The next symptom is titled "Job and Family Problems." While they can be very close cousins to Interpersonal Problems they are usually seen as more definitive in nature. By definitive I mean being late for work, hung over for work, not functioning as expected, being put on probation at work, the loss of jobs, and dysfunction related to getting new jobs. Family issues in this area include the loss of marriages and families, being kept from or avoiding visits with children, and child abuse.

In these days and times few of us need a description of financial problems but this is usually a constant (chronic) problem with the addict. While labeled Chronic the dysfunction

80

is a reaction to being intoxicated or under the influence. These problems can actually be used as a great motivator for change once the addiction is brought into the open. The most prolific cause of problems in this area are not about jobs lost or struggles with employment but instead about the "misappropriation" of resources in order to finance substance use.

Put all these symptoms together and it is no wonder that serious relationship problems exist in the addicted person's life and by extension in the lives of their loved ones. While all these symptoms may seem very closely related they are separated to avoid confusion about cause and effect and to facilitate the user's awareness of the true nature and scope of their problem.

Summarizing

- The Chronic Disease Model of addiction is the evolution of the medial establishment's progress towards understanding and diagnosing addiction.
- Treatment for emotional issues and socio-economic issues are not usually considered or treated under this model.
- Addict behavior is seen as a manifestation of a medical condition caused by excessive use and abuse of a chemical either as the result of genetic predisposition or repeated use.
- While predisposition may quicken the onset of the disease it is not required for the disease state to present. Just like cancer related illnesses, you may have a predisposition to acquiring it but there are still measures to take and behaviors to be avoided that can circumvent becoming ill.
- You can still contract the disease without a family history.

In this model addiction is a purely medical state and as with other Chronic conditions the treatment is usually simple. Once you have it, you have it. Like sugar to the diabetic the drug of addiction must be avoided to retard future progression of the illness. As with all Chronic Disease treatment this usually means getting the user to; abstain from the substance, getting them educated on the disease, to use that information to self-diagnosis, to realize and accept the disease state exists and to then access the available help to treat the permanent condition.

This model is extremely effective if the quality of education leads to proper self-diagnosis, if there is involvement in counseling to extinguish triggers for use, help overcoming obstacles created by use and if 12 step recovery programs are utilized. Like other chronic conditions and illnesses this means a major change in lifestyle and behavior if the diseased person wants to survive and avoid suffering with, and possibly dying from, the malady.

Bio-Psycho-Social Model (Holistic)

The approach of this model may seem obvious by its name but understanding the totality of it may help you more fully connect the dots between all the models already examined. The Bio-Psycho-Social Model is quite simply a culmination of everything we know about addiction being used to treat all the aspects of the illness at the same time. It is easily the most open of all the models: Open to both new research and new ideas.

While many hospitals still operate from a foundation in the medical model they also incorporate the Bio-Psycho-Social Model (BPS) into their treatment planning. Perhaps this is done due to the influence of the mental health profession but it is also done in the hopes of unifying and clarifying the understanding of an addiction diagnosis throughout the health care continuum. In order to have a cohesive framework to communicate across paradigm lines the American Psychological Association has developed the Diagnostic and Statistical Manual (the DSM.) The current rendering is the DSM-V (DSM-IV-TR is the preferred edition for most addiction professionals today.)

The DSM is now accepted as the main reference for all determinations and coding for mental illness in the United States and elsewhere. The book and its coding are used to outline a common base of understanding when communicating across different paradigms and models. When a diagnosis of 303.90 Alcohol Dependence is given (DSM IV), any person in the world working under any paradigm can open the DSM and understand what the assessor is suggesting. The DSM incorporates all aspects of the illness from a B-P-S model approach. The use of the DSM also removes the possibility of the addict or alcoholic knowingly or unknowingly confusing their diagnosis between different treatment programs.

When it was developed the Bio-Psycho-Social model suggested for perhaps the first time, that addiction can have different causes for different people from different environments and socio-economic levels. The Bio-Psycho-Social Model begins by getting the addict detoxified, beginning their education on their illness, providing counseling, getting them introduced into the 12 Step communities and my personal favorite; getting the family supported and guided to aid in their own recovery from the malady. If you look closely at the process I just outlined you will easily see how the different models present themselves across the continuum of care.

Be assured that there is no better approach to addiction "TREATMENT" then to view the problem of addiction as a multifaceted issue with varying causes, conditions and concerns. As we reviewed all the different models of addiction we saw how each narrowly focused model presented numerous deficits, how some even retarded the process and even harmed the addict by not considering all the possible aspects and causes of addiction. This model absolutely believes that all the treatment aspects developed to date can and should be used together to aid the addict in overcoming their malady. It is important to remember that this model does not suggest that we know all we need to know about addiction, quite the opposite in fact: The BPS model encourages more investigation and relies on the therapist or counseling process to determine what is right for the individual, often referred to as clinical judgment (experience).

In the late 80's a phrase "cookie cutter treatment" was coined to bring awareness to the fact that not everyone has the same causes and concerns regarding their addiction and by extension their treatment needs. The phrase is a guidepost of sorts to keep programs from giving the same treatment to everyone who walks through their doors. Sadly this is not always practiced and observed. Your addict may not be a good fit for every program and the dollar value of a treatment program does not correlate to higher success rates (sometimes quite the opposite.) The addict and the program need to be a "good fit" for the best chances of success and for long term recovery to be established. Nothing can replace a seasoned professional, not even a recovery sponsor.

Before we move on I think there is an important awareness you should have to avoid some confusion. While the term addict and alcoholic are the major labels used to describe an agreed upon condition in the public vernacular, the professional counselor or therapist does not diagnose under these terms. The phraseology "Substance Abuser" and "Substance Dependent" are the proper terms of reference in the professional treatment community (DSM-IV). When it is used in these environments the term Addict or Alcoholic does not suggest or imply a negative connotation. It is sometimes suggested in the recovery communities that the terms Addict and Alcoholic are those terms used to self-diagnose, as in "I am an Addict" or "I am an Alcoholic" (More later)

Perhaps the true benefit of the Bio-Psycho-Social Model is that by using a holistic approach to diagnosis we minimize the chances for misdiagnosis and provide a better foundation for comprehensive treatment. By first examining and caring for the physical body we are able to treat emergency needs and conditions including withdrawal and even physical pain issues that might increase the risk of relapse and distract the individual from the learning process ahead of them.

Following the assessment of the physical we arrive at the psychological reasons behind their behaviors and machinations. We often find out that they are dealing with another mental illness, unresolved grief or abuse issues that are too difficult to face without a substance or other legitimate medication. And finally, when viewing issues of the social perspective, are we ignoring the impact of their individual social system on long term recovery? Are they so entrenched in using peers and using/dysfunctional families that a return to those environments would only result in a return to use? These are vital questions.

Since the Bio-Psycho-Social Model truly is our society's current mainstream approach and will most often be the treatment type provided, we will examine it in more detail later, and thereby establish an even greater level of insight into the efforts and needs of the substance user, abuser and dependent.

We learned that the Bio-Psycho-Social Model suggests the following:

- That addiction is caused by more than one factor.
- That each one of these different factors can increase or influence one-another and even further complicate treatment.
- That more than one method of treatment may be required and that multiple efforts and approaches can be applied at the same time.
- That the therapist needs to be educated and experienced in all these facets.

The BPS model allows us to:

- Combine the information attained from an initial comprehensive assessment and to continue to develop our assessment/diagnosis as new information arises.
- It gives options regarding treatment thereby increasing effectiveness and facilitating more positive outcomes.

- Different treatment methods give us many more ways to improve the client's function level thereby improving the addict's success rate and comfort levels.

Addiction is possibly one of the most multifaceted illnesses that can be faced in a health care setting. This care is so difficult that other psych-based caregivers more often than not; refer substance dependents to addictions counselors (people who focus on addiction specifically). This is due to the complex level of skills, experience, and awareness needed to successfully aid the individual in treating himself or herself. These special skills are needed to get them through the myriad of stumbling blocks they will face along the way. The subtle nuances of these stumbling blocks (discussed later) speak to the nature of why it is impossible for the addict to recover on their own. If you are not a professional or a recovering addict yourself (in a 12 Step Program) there is no way you can foresee or predict the obstacles that lie in wait for those persons trying to change these behaviors and overcome or manage their condition.

Part III

Addiction and Mental Illness

Dual Diagnosis

If you love an addict struggling with both addiction and another mental health disorder like Bi-Polar I or II, you have most certainly heard the term Dual Diagnosis. This term is sometimes misinterpreted to suggest that there are two different addictions in place. This is erroneous. This term does not refer to an alcoholic with a cocaine problem: The confusion arises because that state is most often termed Dual Addicted.

The term Dual Diagnosis suggests that an addiction diagnosis is present as well as another mental health diagnosis. For example, an alcohol dependent may also be suffering from Bi-Polar or s/he may have an underlying Personality Disorder. Whichever the combination this greatly complicates the treatment needs of the individual and unfortunately it lessens their success rate when it comes to achieving abstinence.

Where to Start When Both States Exist

There are two perspectives that we should consider when diagnosing a person with a "Dual Diagnosis." Awareness of these 2 states may help many laypersons and professionals alike better understand their loved one's/clients' needs.

- The first scenario is that there are people who have a primary mental illness that has lead to an addiction issue. We categorize this type as a person with a mental illness who has a substance abuse/dependency problem." This is often a result of their attempts to self medicate a

89

problem like depression or mania as well as many others. For example the person who suffers with depression may resort to stimulants to lift their mood or a person with ADD or ADHD may develop a marijuana or alcohol dependency to slow their mind, etc...

- The second category or type; is the substance user that uses for a long enough period of time that a mental illness is brought on by their extended use and the long term practice of unhealthy behaviors. This is often referred to as "a substance dependent with another mental health issue or mental illness." Quite simple, if a person is using a depressant drug like alcohol for a long enough period of time they may (and often do) meet the criteria for depression and therefore may need to be treated accordingly.

This may seem like merely semantics but it has everything to do with WHY THEY USE as well as how they need to be treated if they are to ever successfully arrive at the state of being "clean and sober." Simply put the two types are as follows;

1. A mental health problem that leads to an addiction issue/s
2. An addiction issue that leads to a mental health problem

Under either of the above circumstance the first and primary objective is to get the individual detoxed and stabilized before trying to determine the primary and secondary problems to be treated. I have a simple suggestion to consider when determining which category or condition is presenting. If your loved one has a history of mental illness then get them back on their meds with their prior doctor's direction but be absolutely sure that their doctor is informed (by you) that an addiction issue precipitated the visit.

While confidentiality issues limit what a doctor can tell you they do not limit what or how much information you may give to the counselor or doctor. My advice is to flood the doctor with whatever information you know in regards to the addictive behavior and other treatment processes being undertaken, including all legal and domestic issues.

If your loved one does not have a prior history of mental illness then consider if at all possible holding off the medicating for a mental illness that they might not have. Addicts love the excuse that they are mentally ill. Why? Because then drugs and alcohol aren't the issue and they can return to use once stabilized on their meds. Nothing can be further from the truth, as nearly all drugs prescribed for mental health conditions are rendered useless by the strong mood altering chemicals of abuse and dependency.

Next, I highly suggest that you please consider the feedback and advice of all the people closest to the problem, as their insight is likely to be invaluable. What do I mean by this? I have seen hundreds of cases of people being medicated for non-existent mental illness (distress caused by poor behavior choices like lying and stealing from loved ones is not a mental health condition, it is a behavioral problem). This misdiagnosis and subsequent treatment can almost completely negate the benefits of treatment. One of the reasons is that the mere prescribing of the medication validates their having a problem "other" then addiction, thereby aiding them in DEFOCUSING from treating their addiction problem and increasing their resistance and denial. The best course is reassurance and continued treatment by experienced professionals.

The confusion about primary causes is why it is so hard to treat Dual Diagnosis. While this may not seem like much help my advice is quite simple: If you don't need the meds don't take them. If you do need the meds, take them." A chronic alcoholic who becomes depressed may need a short period of treatment with Anti-depressants to get them through their overwhelming depression caused by fallout from their using and allow them to see the light at the end of the tunnel. The depressive person may not be able to see that light without the help of medication.

With that being said I want to make another point that may seem a little contrary to the one I just made. People with other mental health issues who do not get their dual diagnosis status treated are sometimes considered among the ranks of the chronic relapser. If they have been labeled as such the mere label of Chronic Relapser should be a signal of a deeper under lying condition that needs to be treated. Like I have stated already, addiction is a complex issue that needs to be treated from all the various aspects and paradigms that exist.

Many times dually diagnosed individuals struggle to get clean because their mental health issue is often too overwhelming to face. Recovery is further complicated because their use has been behaviorally reinforced by their having found relief from their mental illness in the substance of abuse. When these patients have their mental health issue stabilized they often experience great success.

For example; a truly depressed person suffering from Bi-Polar issues may find it very difficult to accept or experience the level of hope found by most addicts and alcoholics in 12 Step programs. It's not because they don't get it! It's because the deficit level of helpful neurotransmitters in their brain at the appropriate times doesn't allow them to feel the true elation of personal successes. Additionally, uncovering and facing one's core issues makes it hard to overcome the sadness faced with the uncovering of their behavioral history. The installation of Hope and a positive future outlook is an essential part of a recovery program's success. If a mind cannot be sold the vision of recovery then they won't be able to put out the effort necessary. They will however experience great success if they can honestly share their struggles with both professionals and other 12 step program members. There are many dual diagnosis programs available to help with these struggles.

This book isn't about medicating or not medicating. It's about understanding WHY THEY USE and how to have success in overcoming the problems of, and increasing the understanding of, addiction. Personally, I struggle with the idea of using drugs to treat a drug problem. Professionally I have tried to avoid having my clients medicated because I want them to experience the full benefits and joys of their recovery efforts without giving the benefits of their change over to the medication.

I practice the above perspective because I don't want my clients thinking at their one-year recovery anniversary that their medication is what facilitated their accomplishment. (Unfortunately this is sometimes not a luxury.) After more than 25 years of exposure to the recovery communities I can promise you that when fully applied, the processes of 12 step recovery programs are extremely effective for all but the severely mentally ill; provided the individual can be honest with themselves and follow the directions that are clearly outlined. The author of the book "Alcoholics Anonymous" (William Griffith Wilson) believed himself to be suffering from a Bi-Polar illness. Not only did he overcome the malady with the spiritual principles they set in place, he also helped to create a program of action to address addiction that is seen as 100% effective when closely followed.

Yes, medication can help addicts to experience success but the gains will always be diminished at the cost of their self-esteem and self-efficacy. This is a difficult choice and should be decided only after serious consultation with a psychiatrist experienced in addiction medicine. The costs and benefits of both approaches should be weighed carefully. (Note, most psychiatrists will medicate you if you pay for a visit.)

If the user is still struggling to be happy after some success attaining time clean and sober, without medication, (one to two years) then I reconsider medication needs and help them to find informed and competent professional help. If they can't grasp the hope they should gleam from the programs and their outlook is negative I will pay close attention and consider a referral.

Definition of Mental Disorder (DSM-IV-TR)

The following is a more technical definition but I want you to have some more awareness and insight into the professional language used in the DSM-IV-TR to describe the state often referred to as a "mental illness" or a mental health dis-order.

A mental health disorder is conceptualized as a clinically significant behavioral or psychological syndrome or pattern that occurs in an individual and that is associated with the present distress (painful symptoms) or disability (impairment in one or more areas of functioning) or with a significantly increased risk of suffering death, pain, disability, or an important loss of freedom.

Even as a clinician that definition can seem a little wordy or confusing. Basically, what is being suggested is that a "mental illness" is an illness that results in thinking and behaviors that cause life problems and emotional discomfort. These problems can be life threatening or just cause major distress. The condition leads to a way of living, which leaves the individual missing out on many of life's most rewarding experiences. Also note the use of the term "present." A mental disorder is seen as a snapshot in time. The DSM shies away from permanently labeling an individual as a mental illness, as in "he's bi-polar." It instead references the individual as suffering from a bi-polar condition but only because of the information provided during the time of diagnosis. A person may be easily misdiagnosed as suffering from a Bi-polar condition if they fail to report to the assessor that they are addicted to cocaine or some other drug.

Diagnostic Criteria

So how does a professional arrive at a diagnosis? Diagnostic Criteria are simply a type of benchmark used to form a diagnosis. These "markers" indicate what symptoms must be present (and for how long) in order to qualify for a diagnosis (called inclusion criteria) as well as those symptoms that must not be present (called exclusion criteria) in order for an individual to qualify for a particular diagnosis. They provide a simplified compact encapsulated description of what constitutes each specific disorder. The use of diagnostic criteria has been shown to increase diagnostic reliability (i.e., likelihood that different clinicians will assign the same diagnosis and by extension, treatment). The criteria are meant to only be used as a guideline to be supported and formed by clinical judgment (the professional's experience) and are not meant to be used in a cookbook fashion for treatment.

You will see the following parameter more than once in the DSM: *"Addiction is part of the exclusion criteria for almost every mental illness."* The clinician is directed to RO (rule out) the existence of a general medical condition and the possibility of a substance induced cause before applying any diagnosis other than a substance use disorder. Why? Because as I stated earlier, the symptoms of a substance dependent state can mimic other mental health issues (ie. Depression brought on by alcohol abuse or dependence and mania brought on by stimulant use).

Substance Related Disorders

Once again; I am providing this information because if you have a loved one who requires treatment you will need a foundation of understanding to grasp the process they will go through. This process has, as mentioned before, many stumbling blocks and pitfalls along the way.

When used in a clinical setting a substance is defined as a drug of abuse, which can also include prescription drugs, nicotine, caffeine and alcohol. THE DSM has grouped the substances into 11 classes in alphabetical order. Some share significant and similar features.

The substance related disorders are grouped as follows:
- Substance Use Disorders (Abuse & Dependency)
- Substance Induced Disorders
    - Substance Intoxication
    - Substance Withdrawal
    - Substance-Induced Delirium
    - Substance-Induced Persisting Dementia
    - Substance-Induced Persisting Amnestic Dis.
    - Substance-Induced Psychotic Disorder
    - Substance-Induced Mood Disorder
    - Substance-Induced Anxiety Disorder
    - Substance-Induced Induced Sexual Dysfunction
    - Substance-Induced Sleep Disorder

(If you paid close attention to the list you noticed that it suggested some major psychiatric conditions caused by substance use, even psychotic episodes.)

As mentioned before in the reading and further on, drugs are put into classes or families based on their effect on the human body. The Drug Classes in the DSM-IV-TR are as follows; Sedative, Hypnotic, or Anxiolytic/Alcohol, Amphetamine, Caffeine, Cannabis, Cocaine, Hallucinogens, Inhalant/Volatile, Nicotine, Opioid, Phencyclidine, Polysubstance and Other/Unknown (for new drugs.)

In order for a clinician (or layperson) to determine whether the user is an abuser or a substance dependent they must first establish an understanding as to what is meant by the terms "Substance Withdrawal and Tolerance." They must also understand how each of the drug classes' present with specific "symptoms" of withdrawal. More simply speaking they need to know how withdrawal and tolerance present (in symptomology) for each class/type of a drug. For example; did you know that a common symptom of marijuana/cannabis withdrawal is extreme irritability and a low frustration tolerance? If a family member brings a young person to my office and I notice a low frustration tolerance then I might investigate marijuana use, especially if the family makes statements like "He used to be such a happy kid." I may even have a urine screen done to establish a baseline of truth. KNOW THIS FOR CERTAIN: People who are not using will always consent to a test, if for no other reason than to prove someone else wrong. If they refuse then I operate as if a positive test has been achieved. (More later)

I believe that by learning some of these signs you will better understand some of the possible behaviors that a loved one is presenting and you will thereby better understand that they are acting that way because of their withdrawal syndrome. They are not acting that way because you raised them wrong or because you don't love them the right way. Their withdrawal causes them to act in specific ways and that while you may be the target of their accusations you are not the cause of their discomfort. They are merely subconsciously defending the substance from being the cause of the problem because they have learned that re-administration of the chemical will actually bring relief. THAT IS EMOTIONAL DEPENDENCY ON A SUBSTANCE. This knowledge should also help you determine for yourself if your concerns for their physical safety are warranted.

Withdrawal

Withdrawal Defined (DSM et al)

- The development of a substance-specific syndrome due to the cessation of (or reduction in) substance use that has been heavy and prolonged. (It is the body's reaction to what happens when they can't get enough of their drug to maintain the body's false, drug induced, homeostasis.)

- The substance-specific syndrome causes clinically significant distress or impairment in social, occupational, or other important areas of functioning (They are not meeting their responsibility due to their "not feeling well." This includes hangover related lost time from work etc...)

- The symptoms are not due to a general medical condition and are not better accounted for by another mental disorder. (This basically says there is no cause beyond the substance use and its apparent withdrawal symptomology. This is when it is crucial to determine which of the two types of Dual Diagnosis is presenting.)

As suggested in the criteria above, withdrawal occurs when the user's administration of the substance is either reduced or stopped. Because of the cessation of use, the body's false homeostasis in upset and the body reacts due to the absence of a chemical the body has become dependent on. This is associated with the more severe substance level diagnosis of Substance Dependency and not merely Substance Abuse. The Dependency diagnosis is in essence the true state referred to in mainstream society as alcoholism or addiction.

Withdrawal causes individuals to have more cravings for their drug of choice, which results in a need/desire to re-administer the substance, hence dependence. When the substance is used to treat the discomfort of withdrawal the need for the substance becomes perversely reinforced (Behavioral conditioning). This process creates the false belief that the drug is required in order to find relief thereby increasing the level of emotional need for the substance. This reinforcing is perhaps the greatest hurdle or stumbling block encountered when substance abstinence is sought.

To understand withdrawal and in order to keep it simple, most of the symptoms of withdrawal are the opposite of those effects experienced and observed during intoxication or use of the chemical. Cocaine speeds your heart rate up and lifts up you mood when you use it so the crash and withdrawal are usually just that, a crash resulting in reduced energy, lethargy and dysphoria.

Heroin/opiate addicts become most uncomfortable when experiencing withdrawal because the drug that once removed all pain, calmed them down to a state of sleep and created "nervous system sedation" now (during withdrawal) ignites every nerve center in their body, forcing the overly rested nervous system to become hypersensitive to all pain and discomfort. Is it really any wonder that the addicted resorts back to the drug for relief? Once they do use the chemical to treat the symptoms of withdrawal the appropriately named "Vicious Cycle" begins all over again. (As an aside, the term "kick the habit" was originally a descriptive term for opiate withdrawal. As the addict's system withdrew from the chemical their knees would draw up towards their bodies, then in a mini spasm both legs would kick straight out away from their chest. This was most often experienced while lying on a bathroom floor (hence, kick the habit).

Acute Withdrawal

A more highly variable range of signs and symptomology characterizes acute withdrawal. Remember; "Acute Conditions" come on fast, are severe but run a simple course. The condition is not a permanent aspect of the body's function like chronic conditions are.

These acute symptoms include somewhat moderate levels of; sweating, tachycardia, hypertension, tremors, and anxiety, to more serious consequences including seizures and delirium tremens. The etiology of acute withdrawal has been hypothesized to involve one or more neuronal and hormonal systems of the body. This process is worsened because the body is often experiencing a deficit of these chemicals due to poor diet choices and the malnutrition states usually experienced by the addicted body/person. While some drug withdrawals are life threatening and are a physical manifestation of the body going into shock they all run a prescribed and predictable course of symptoms and time frames. If your addict seems to be experiencing unreasonably long periods of detoxification then they may have re-administered the drug when you were not watching.

Protracted Withdrawal

Protracted withdrawal is a term used to describe a type of withdrawal event that is often a major stumbling block for the substance dependent person. This phenomenon is also often referred to as protracted abstinence syndrome, late withdrawal or even a "dry drunk." The professional medical community is still examining this complicated issue. The person suffering from this state/condition is usually caught off-guard as they rarely know that what they are experiencing is a common and treatable event in the recovery process. The addict often becomes very disillusioned by the notion that they are not getting away from the drug's hold over them. They begin to believe that they will never feel better than they currently do. They quickly become convinced that they will never be able to exist without experiencing strong cravings, no matter how long they remain clean and sober. They enter into a depressive and confused state because they don't have an understanding of what they are experiencing. Twelve-Step Recovery Programs are amazing at remedying this problem.

Pharmacological treatment (drugs to help get them through the process) has been hampered by the lack of consistent agreement on distinctive signs and symptoms and the duration of the abstinence syndromes. Giving the addict a drug to treat a drug condition is difficult to justify when not obviously needed. The problem arises when certain segments of the treatment community start to suggest that every addict get the treatment to avoid the "possible" stumbling block of protracted withdrawal. This process requires the insights and attention of a professional clinician and not simply another recovering addict. The recovery programs merely provide the essential ingredients of HOPE and SUPPORT not available in a prescription.

The purported symptoms of Abstinence Syndrome include: Anxiety, Irritability, Hostility, Depression, Insomnia, Catastrophizing, Fatigue, and stronger cravings then experienced in recent weeks. Obviously one could argue that anyone trying to recover from an addiction would and even should experience these symptoms. Recent research has suggested that a "Kindling effect" may contribute to symptoms of protracted withdrawal, which leads to cravings and the eventual relapse. Kindling is seen as a type of mounting disillusionment with recovery, a slow building of negative attitudes and catastrophizing or awfullizing their feelings about a possible comfortable future in recovery.

This may be a big factor in Why They Use and Use, again. More research and then education about those findings is certainly needed.

Physiological Addiction

We covered the basics of "Physiological Addiction" earlier while discussing the medical model. Briefly it is a condition where the body becomes accustomed to the presence of a chemical. (Ever had a caffeine addiction?) The body has created a new state or level of homeostasis that now incorporates the drug into its existence. The body reacts to maintain homeostasis and thereby either raises or lowers the corresponding Central Nervous System thresholds like heart rate and blood pressure to adjust to this change. When the chemical is not present we have the previously aforementioned state called Withdrawal as the body attempts to adjust. When the chemical is removed, the body can respond either quickly or slowly depending on the chemical's half-life (how long to takes to metabolize half the chemical in the body). Death can result in those individuals who go through severe withdrawal due to their Physiological Addiction and the body's inability to transition smoothly from one state to another.

Conditioning/Conditioned Response

As we read about in the previous chapter on the Behavioral Model of addiction, conditioning is the result of an association between one action or event and another action or event with the anticipated event being either rewarding (positively reinforcing) or causing discomfort (negatively reinforcing.) A good experience reinforces the behavior and a negative one extinguishes the behavior. Either way there is a behavioral change in order to resolve some form of anxiety. This "learned behavior pattern" and its response are rooted in the limbic system's processes of fight or flight, the home of all stress and all reward. The reinforcing of the behavior is also affected by the amount of time between the behavior or action and the reward or negative stimuli. This is also true when it comes to substances of abuse. The faster a substance enters the body, (the sooner the gratification or reduction in anxiety) the stronger the emotional attachment is to the chemical process/behavior.

Once conditioning has been established it can be imprinted into the individual's psyche so strongly that any future return to the pattern re-ignites all the previous conditioning and by extension the emotional attachments (much like connecting with an old lover). In regards to cigarette or nicotine addiction, this is why having even "just one" is a bad idea. Total abstinence is the only way to avoid regenerating the emotional bond of the addict for their substance of choice.

Understanding the DSM IV
Diagnostic Criteria
Abuse and Dependency

As promised earlier, the following data is a further look into the DSM IV Diagnostic Criteria as it relates to addiction. It should still be considered brief and by no means a complete summary of the various aspects of addictive disease as it is presented in the Diagnostic and Statistical Manual, forth addition with Technical Revisions (DSM-IV-TR). Once again the DSM is the most widely used source of addiction coding in the United States and most of the world. The DSM is the mechanism by which counselors, addiction professionals, psychologists, psychiatrists, clinical social workers and insurance companies standardize and agree upon diagnosis.

When trying to understand and determine the severity of your loved one's condition you will find the following information to be important and helpful benchmarks for you to consider. The following specific criteria are used to determine if either a Substance Abuse state or a Substance Dependent state is present. You may find it easier to replace the terms Abuse and Dependency with the more common terms drug problem and drug addiction. (I do not support or endorse DSM V changes.)

Substance Abuse Criteria from the DSM IV-TR

Substance Abuse is a maladaptive pattern of substance use leading to clinically significant impairment or distress, as manifested by one (or more) of the following, occurring within a 12-month period (try checking them off if they apply to your loved one. The more that apply, the greater the severity)

- Recurrent substance use resulting in a failure to fulfill major role obligations at work, school, or home (e.g., poor work or homework performance related to substance use; substance-related absences, suspensions, or expulsions from school; neglect of children or the household)

- Recurrent substance use in situations in which it is physically hazardous (e.g., driving an automobile or operating a machine when impaired by substance use). (This could also be considered for the caregivers of young children, as their being intoxicated so frequently that it manifests into a form of neglect.)
- Recurrent substance-related legal problems (e.g., arrests for substance-related disorderly conduct, DWI, drinking in public, possession charges, etc…)
- Continued substance use despite having persistent or recurrent social or interpersonal problems caused or exacerbated by the effects of the substance (e.g., arguments with spouse about consequences of intoxication, physical fights, arguments with co workers about performance, etc…)

"Substance Dependency" is the more severe form of "addictive" illness. Once the criteria/symptoms have been met for substance dependence for this same class of a drug (Alcohol = Seditives,) the diagnosis would be given for dependence and not substance abuse. As we have already learned the key identifiers that separate substance abuse and substance dependency are the existence of tolerance and withdrawal.

DSM IV View of Substance Abuse Explored Further

As stated above: The diagnosis for abuse does not consider tolerance or withdrawal or a pattern of compulsive use but instead focuses more directly on the harmful consequences of repeated use and the failings or shortcomings that result from that pattern of use. Because Dependence on many drugs can occur quickly "Substance Abuse" is more likely to be identified in individuals who have more recently started taking the specific substance. With this in mind it is still possible for some individuals to continue to have substance related adverse social consequences and problems for many years without evidence of physical dependence (tolerance or withdrawal).

As an interesting aside the DSM directs the reader to not apply these criteria to caffeine and nicotine, mostly because tolerance and withdrawal happen much more rapidly with caffeine and nicotine and the social issues identified in the abuse criteria actually take longer to present. If cigarettes were illegal these consequences and abuse criteria might present much more clearly in regards to Nicotine Addiction.

One should be careful to not use the term "Substance Abuse" as a synonym for "use," "misuse," or "hazardous use." Substance Abuse is a diagnosis and not a reference to addiction per say. Some people see the Ab-use as Ab-normal patterns of Use, Ab-normal-use = Abuse.

DSM-IV Criteria for Substance Dependence

(See above for Substance Abuse Criteria)

Substance Dependence is seen as a maladaptive pattern of substance use, leading to "clinically significant impairment" or distress, as manifested by three (or more) of the following, occurring at any time in the same 12-month period: (Remember to check them off, each number counts as one)

1. Tolerance as defined by either of the following:

   - A need for markedly increased amounts of the substance to achieve intoxication or a desired effect (they used to have two beers now they're having 6)

   - Markedly diminished effect with continued use of the same amount of the substance (they might not be using more but they seem to be less effected, it's hard to tell if they've used. This is sometimes termed Behavioral Tolerance.)

2. Withdrawal, as manifested by either of the following:

   - The characteristic withdrawal syndrome for the substance is observed (typical for the drug, recall that many withdrawal symptoms are the opposite of the drugs effect, stimulant users get tired during withdrawal, opiate addicts get fidgety, sedative/alcohol users get anxious)

   - The same (or a closely related) substance is taken to relieve or avoid withdrawal symptoms (an alcoholic uses benzodiazepines (valium) or a heroin addict might use pain killers like codeine/opiates to stop the body's reaction to cessation.)

3. The substance is often taken in larger amounts or over a longer period of time than was intended. ("I only

stopped by for one beer then I got to talking with the guys," "Oh my God look what time it is!" The problem is not that they forgot the time but that they have failed to fulfill other obligations.)

4. There is a persistent desire or unsuccessful efforts to cut down or control substance use (failed attempt to stop or a currently held belief that they should stop.)

5. A great deal of time is spent in activities necessary to obtain the substance (e.g., visiting multiple doctors or driving long distances to get the drug), this can also be large amounts of time to actually use and administer the substance.)

6. Important social, occupational, or recreational activities are given up or reduced because of substance use. (They can't drink at the school so they avoid school activities. They stop going to movies, or don't want to go to the in-laws because they can't consume alcohol the way they want while there, etc.)

7. The substance use is continued despite knowledge of having persistent or recurrent physical or psychological problems that are likely to have been caused or exacerbated by the substance (e.g., current cocaine use despite recognition of cocaine-induced depression, or continued drinking despite recognition that an ulcer is made worse by alcohol consumption, etc...)

How did they do? How many did you check off? Three or more? I think it is important that you remember that these criteria should be viewed by the layperson as being an indicator of severity. Even one of the above can become a major problem and as with all substance use at any level the possibility of sudden death can occur. Each of the criteria should be taken very seriously, and viewed as serious warning signs all by themselves.

Substance Induced Disorders

Substance Induced Disorders are the types of mental illnesses that are directly caused by substance use, abuse and dependency. These conditions do not exist prior to substance use and often do not exist without the presence of the substance in the body. As mentioned previously these are emotional issues, which are caused by or brought on by substance use. A substance abuse problem that causes a mental illness can occur during substance abuse levels of use but are most frequently associated with substance dependence. The following are a variety of symptoms that are characteristic of other mental disorders. These complications go beyond the scope of this book but I thought it might be helpful to mention them in case your addict is diagnosed with a similar mental illness while being treated for their substance problem. (Pay special attention to the diagnosis after the word induced. If your addict is diagnosed with anyone of these conditions separate from their addiction, be sure to inform the assessor of the substance problem because it must be given priority.)

- Substance-Induced Delirium
- Substance-Induced Persisting Dementia
- Substance-Induced Persisting Amnestic Disorder (memory)
- Substance-Induced Psychotic Disorder
- Substance-Induced Mood Disorder
- Substance-Induced Anxiety Disorder
- Substance-Induced Sexual Dysfunction
- Substance-Induced Sleep Disorder

- Hallucinogen Persisting Perception Disorder (flashbacks or hallucinations, including audio)

A detailed history is required before making a diagnosis of any mental health problem. When possible all additional outside sources of information should be accessed. As a previous owner of an assessment and intervention company, I can assure you that the assessment process is the most important aspect of any treatment agenda. Over the years I have found it helpful to sometimes have one entity diagnose and another treat the diagnosis. This can limit the possibility of a diagnosis based on a bias, as programs often over diagnose the issues they most frequently treat. Before any mental health diagnosis is confirmed all medical conditions must be ruled out first and foremost. Physical examinations and the findings of laboratory tests can be extremely helpful and spare addicts and families' needless suffering.

Part IV
Addict Denial

When it comes to the topic of denial it's quite possible that most of us would not be nearly as cognizant of the word had the addict not popularized the term through their seemingly purposeful refusal to see the error of their ways and admit to their problem. There is a saying in the recovery community; "Denial is not a river in Egypt." The statement pokes fun at the depths of denial the addict experiences, to the point that they don't even hear or recognize the word denial. The 12 step programs' first step speaks to admitting the problem as the primary condition for recovery. This acknowledgement is the crux of any possible or potential change for the addict. Without a personal revelation about the severity of the problem the hopes for change are short lived at best.

Let's take a closer look at the dynamics surrounding a person who becomes so confused and distracted by their need to use that they can no longer see what is so apparent to everyone around them. This is a person who refuses to acknowledge their own problem so adamantly that their significant others begin to take this refusal to see the obvious, as a personal affront. Another saying goes; "The addict is always the last person to know." This saying suggests it has already become blatantly obvious to everyone else around him or her. By this time their families have stopped calling them, their bosses let them go or reassigned them, their lovers have moved on and eventually even the legal system has to do for them what they "won't" do for themselves. Somewhat surprisingly the addict is still convinced that they're just having a run of bad luck. Before we proceed with a specific focus on addict denial let's examine how it is possible for the human mind to become self-deceived.

Self-Deception

Denial is actually self-deception. Before we can understand self-deception we must first define deception. Deception is what many of us most often term a lie and it is usually between two or more people. Popular understanding of "other-deception" (not self deception) says that in order for deception to occur there must first exist:

a) An intentional plan to mislead or to alter the truth and;

b) That there must actually be a held belief on the part of the deceived, as a result of the information given. (Barnes 95).

Here is an example: If I tell you that California is on the East Coast and I believe it, and you believe me, then I have not deceived you. I have instead misled you because I have no intent to trick you. If I knowingly tell you the East Coast when I know it's the West Coast, and you then believe what I have told you then I have deceived you. There has to be intention on my part (to mislead you) and belief on yours (being California is on the East Coast). These two states or conditions must exist in order for other deception to have occurred.

When this scenario is limited to one person and one mind the question then arises about whether or not it is possible for an individual to purposely deceive/convince themselves of something they don't initially believe. Changes in the notion held must take place. This means that the individual has to adopt a notion contrary to the previous notion held without recognizing that the process or change in belief is taking place. They have to eventually believe what they are telling themselves. They have to purposely work toward attaining a notion contrary to what evidence is telling them.

Because of popular Drug Education policies in the US all children educated here start with the notion that drugs are bad or harmful. "Just say no!" Before a shift in notion can occur and in order for this to happen a person must be able to first hold two contrasting ideas in their head at the same time. This is actually not hard to do and we do this all the time.

A very simplified example of holding two contrasting ideas in one's mind would be the contrasting between hot and cold. If we were to put our hand under a faucet that was set in the middle range of hot and cold and we were then asked to choose either hot or cold to describe the temperature we would be holding two contrasting ideas in our head at the same time and trying to determine which one to choose based on the evidence that we literally had at hand.

If we were then told that we would be given a large sum of money if it felt more cool then warm, we would naturally look for evidence to substantiate our now "desired" condition or belief, even if we originally found the water to be warm. Thus a notion not yet held. We might posit a rationalization like; "water on the skin is always cooler once the air hits it" or "its cooler then the air temperature" etc… We may even wait to pull our hand from the water to feel it at its coolest.

When an anxiety factor is incorporated into the mix of any objective decision then resolution to that anxiety is given priority over right and wrong, over truth and reality. The individual thus adapts and sustains a notion, which is naturally sought as a means of resolving the anxiety. They want the large sum of money. What this means is that there is a gain to be had if the notion is adopted. Just like in "other" deception, there is a motive.

Resolution to the anxiety eventually becomes the priority, not right and wrong. Our brains have developed and are

115

prioritized to feeling better by reducing anxiety. In this case the anxiety is associated with the possibly of not getting the money. The truth takes a back seat to the potential financial gain. Our motive is to reduce the anxiety associated with missing our chance to gain the cash. If enough evidence exists to substantiate our desired belief then we are on our way to adopting the "desired notion." If enough evidence can validate the desired "right" answer, then the anxiety leaves us or is dissipated. We get paid because the water really is cool! This reduction in anxiety is the engine that fuels the denial of the addict.

A curious thing also happens during this shift in perception and belief. Since we are not interested in substantiating the undesired belief we now begin to conveniently forget the evidence that would support the contrary outcome. We remember the water as being cooler than it really was. In Deception Theory this concept is often referred to as "Walling Off." We create a list of things to support our desired outcome and "unwittingly" begin to forget the arguments to the contrary. Once again we are on our way to believing what we want or even "need" to believe.

Another example: The legal system is an interesting structure that is designed in such a way that each party can focus strictly on "their side" of the two choices of an issue, usually guilty or not guilty. The belief is that an impartial jury or judge can balance the facts once given an accurate list of "all" the pros and cons of an argument. Picture if you will the Scales of Justice. Just like in the court trial the believed victor is the side with the biggest list, the side that tips the scales. Judges and jurors become convinced by the preponderance of evidence available or "allowed." Our "judgments" about personal and emotional issues work in just this same way. (As an interesting aside the statue of Justice is blindfolded.)

Returning to the addict: The substance abuser is almost always attempting to reduce their anxiety. This is how they got into trouble in the first place. We might say they are predisposed to self-deception because they have over trained their brains to reduce or avoid anxiety. This reduction in anxiety (reduction in stress) is in essence the benefit they first came to enjoy early in their use. As they continue to use, much of the anxiety and stress they experience is actually caused by the substance use itself. As long as the chemical is taken the substance still works as an anxiety "solution," regardless of the initial cause or stimuli responsible for the stress. Even if the stress is caused by the substance use the substance still resolves the stress and reduces the associated discomfort. (More on the limbic system later)

The stress of life and the stress of using often become so great for the addicted that a stronger mood altering drug, or larger doses of the drug used, are eventually the only thing that seemingly gives the user the "needed relief." The evolution of self-deception for the addict is contained in that very descriptive term; "needed relief."

On the one hand they are deceived that their discomfort must always be, or "needs to be" relieved, this is not true. They also have to believe that their drug of choice actually works to achieve this solution. As mentioned above and quite to the contrary, the true source of discomfort for most chemical dependents is actually their substance use. They become so deceived that the actual cause of 90% of their problems is now believed to be their only solution.

This phenomenon is precisely why the addict begins to use more of a drug or transitions to harder drugs. They need more help as the effectiveness of the initial drug or amount used to overcome the rationale fails to aid in their "denial of their addiction." In recent popular vernacular it would suggest that they would have to have and do have a "willing suspension of disbelief," hence, self-deception.

Part V

Why They Use and Use and Use
STRESS

What about It?

An old comedian used to say; "If you had my wife you'd drink too." This quote isn't about wives it's about stress. As long as addicts are experiencing stressful conditions the addict will default to use in order to seek relief from that stress. Not because they think it's a good idea but instead because they have become conditioned to believe that the drug can bring relief.

Stress is a part of the human condition and it will always occur. The addict has reached a point where s/he can no longer find a solution beyond the substance; when left to their own devices they hit the default button and use. One of the reasons why this dilemma presents is because they have stopped using their intellect to resolve their problems. This has resulted because their repeated use has led them to believe that the only thing working to resolve their discomfort is their chemical of choice. By this point they have even eliminated some other mood altering chemicals as possible solutions and have now arrived at a preferred drug of choice. We can earnestly say they are self-deceived; they are in denial that other solutions exist. On their own, they can no longer find anything else to address or resolve their discomfort.

This "end-state" is the mental and emotional crux of the disease of addiction. This is why they are so defensive when in withdrawal and why they often feel threatened or cornered.

119

When we threaten their chemical we are threatening to take away their only solution to discomfort. This is why they either want to fight with you or take flight and run away. How many times have you heard; "I don't need this....?"

Unfortunately for the addict the stress they experience when confronted about their addiction often overwhelms them and thereby creates the "stressed state" that they treat with the substance itself. This is a very vicious cycle. The solution has really become the cause. Unfortunately the people who most want the addict to quit cause more stress by threatening the addicts supposed "stress cure." In order for the addict to give up the drug and abstain, solutions have to be offered that address the mountain of stress created during active use and to provide a method to replace the supposed benefit of the substance as a stress reducer.

Quitting use and getting through an addiction is an extremely stress-full period. Facing the wreckage of the past is overwhelming. Asking them to stop using is more severe then asking a person who likes to run or jog to stop and to find something else to do instead of their favorite exercise. Perhaps a similar contrast would be like asking a religious figure (Priest, Monk, Imam, Yogi or Rabbi) to give up their religion. Seriously, take a second and think about that, what is their God?

Lets consider an example: An addict gets arrested does a night in jail, gets released the next morning and is now confronted with the anxiety of a pending trial, jail time, more financial commitments to their lawyer, angered family and even the possible loss of a job. The one coping mechanism that they used (their drug) is not only no longer an option, but is actually the cause of the problem. Couple this with the shame of the above event and repairing the wreckage created by using and the stress quickly becomes overwhelming; 99% of the time they will use, and take further flight into their addiction, escalating the problem even more. A vicious cycle for sure.

But wait! The piling on has not stopped yet. The significant others around the addict want so much to have an impact on the addict, that they begin to bombard them with information about their past misdeeds. A sort of; "while I got your attention!" At this juncture the stress of honestly looking at the wreckage of their addiction will be much more than they can handle and it will be too much for quite some time. This is one of the reasons many treatment programs restrict family contact for the first couple days.

Many family members only think they have to wait until the addict has been initially detoxed to begin their personal cathartic battle to reinforce the addicts need to remain clean & sober. I promise you this is not the time. We are not letting them off the hook. Overwhelming them will only result in relapse. We must give the change a chance to happen.

A MOMENT ABOUT YOU

The addict's dilemma spelled out in this section is the very reason I wrote this book. Someone needs to help you (the loved ones of an addict) through your own recovery process. You have become emotionally sick too and must now get your own emotional house in order. The alcoholic is like an emotional fog machine and you have gotten lost in that fog. Your recovery and growth must occur separate from theirs. Your recovery is not contingent on theirs. It is not necessary for them to change for you to heal. At this point, today, you must begin your own process to clear away any wreckage caused in your environment, in your head, and in your heart.

Deal with It: The Limbic System Doesn't Get it

Increased levels of stress are difficult for everyone. More functional individuals learn how to handle stress in healthier ways. But what exactly is stress and why do we feel it. Stress, as it is most often referred to, is really born of fear or an impending threat to one's survival. The type of fear that we call stress, is usually not thought of as the type that threatens our physical well-being per say, but in modern society it is instead seen as a threat to our level of peace and security (most often financial security). This division between types of stress is an erroneous one. The human body and brain do not know the difference between types or causes of stress. A stress "REACTION" is a physiological event. While high levels of stress are known to precipitate many different illnesses, stress in its most basic state exists to keep us alive. A "stress reaction" is the body preparing itself for either fight or flight.

All animals have stress because all animals, like us, have a limbic system. It is the limbic system that is the home of the fight or flight responses of all animals. It is one of the oldest parts of the organic brain. Fight or flight is therefore one of the most basic emotional responses of any type of organic brain. The limbic system is frequently referenced to as the lizard brain. This reference is due to its being the locus of control and function of the reptile. Eat and don't get eaten. We once had this very stress and it was once our only stress.

The limbic system exists for one reason and one reason only, to sustain life. The limbic system houses many of the functions related to animal survival. It protects us against physical threats to physical well-being, it reminds us when to eat, and attracts us to that perfect mate so we can have that enjoyably reinforcing thing called sex, which in turn tricks us into having offspring. This is believed by most biologists to be the reason why it is in fact, enjoyable. It's enjoyable so that we will keep doing it and perpetuate the species (survival of the species.) Addicts keep using because using has tricked the limbic system into believing that using will aid in survival. It is not a rational process.

If we go back to human evolution in the plains of Africa we can easily understand the origin and function of the human limbic system. What stress did the cave man or the man in the bush have? They didn't have bill collectors, landlords, taxmen, or even husbands and wives as we know them today. Their lives were simple. Get something to eat and don't get eaten while you're doing it. These guys/gals lived in their limbic systems. It is believed that the early human brain was once much more like those of reptile brains then we may want to believe. We certainly didn't have any mastery over making distinctions between our needs and wants.

Imagine the first man that went out hunting in the bush (perhaps with friends) and let's say they came across a Saber-Tooth Tiger. Early man's brain gave him only two choices, to fight and have dinner or to take flight and avoid being dinner. We can presume that at some point man thought he could vanquish the Tiger and his friends surely watched as he was killed and eaten. The next guy that met the Tiger recalled the experience of his departed friend (conditioning) and took flight or we might say, ran like hell. While this may have been a single event the trauma of the event left a deep-seated imprint, exactly like post traumatic stress disorder, PTSD. Imagine seeing your friend eaten by a purple dinosaur, would you be worried when you saw the next one.

Relapse and the Limbic System

Without getting into too much of human physiology our brain has two major areas/parts. The first area/part is sometimes referred to as the neocortex. It is located in the front part of the skull or head. The neocortex receives and stores information for decision-making and remembering; the higher level functions of the brain. The second area but a much more primary part of the brain is generalized as the mid-brain or the limbic system. The limbic system area of the brain controls all the automatic systems (Autonomic Nervous System, ANS) of the body as well as the survival reactions related to outside threats (stressors). Most germane to our discussion are those systems responsible for the survival responses of "fight or flight" contained within the Limbic System.

When you feel threatened, the responses of fight or flight act as a protective response that tells you to either defend yourself or run away. It prepares the body for this by dumping large doses of various hormones and neurotransmitters into the cardiovascular system. This is done to provide you with and prepare you for, the following physical demands that will be needed for either task of fight or flight. It constricts the cardio vascular system, raises blood pressure and provides adrenalin, not for a "feeling" but instead for a physical event.

This Stress Reaction (or feeling as we refer to it today) was strictly created to save our lives from direct threats. Unfortunately for us our social evolution has created scenarios that are inescapable and thereby leave us with lasting levels of stress hormones that are not extinguished/resolved; like mortgage payments and even worries about loved ones. These are situations that cannot be powered through with pure physicality or escaped (by running.) The evolution of our limbic system has yet to find a way to process and resolve these events without the physical exertion of fight or flight.

It is unfortunate for us that the limbic system does not have the benefit of memory like the neocortex. It is purely a conditioned response to perceived stimuli. The limbic system doesn't know the difference between yesterday and 30 years ago. That's an issue of memory. It is strictly concerned with being alive right now. This explains why childhood traumas can still trigger us today. It's because the Limbic system does not know that the event was 30 years ago. It has evolved and is designed to protect us from the Saber Tooth Tiger regardless of when we saw him last.

It is the limbic system that is most affected by our life and death experiences. The limbic system can be negatively programmed through traumatic experiences, such as growing up in a dangerous environment or a dysfunctional family. It is programmed by tragic events like being raped, robbed or involved in a terrible accident. Post Traumatic Stress Disorder is a condition of the Limbic System.

As discussed earlier, the body dumps chemicals in the system to prepare the individual for fight or flight, sometimes known as a stress reaction. When a mood-altering drug of abuse in introduced into the system during a stress reaction those chemicals trick the limbic system into thinking that the fight or the flight activity has occurred. The system believes that the threat has been resolved. Since the limbic system doesn't have a memory or since it doesn't conduct rational thought it cannot tell itself or remind itself that the threat is still there. The limbic system has been bluffed by the false resolution of the stressful stimulus. It becomes programmed to believe that the mood-altering chemical is a newly discovered solution to the threat of survival. The limbic system is for all intents and purposes,

DUMB! The altering of the Central Nervous System (by either speeding up a body system or by slowing down a body system) mimics the physical event of running or fighting. Thus the Limbic system becomes falsely convinced that a resolution to the problem of stress has been resolved and that the body can now return to its normal pre-stressed state.

Other behaviors that provide us with pleasure through neuro-chemical reward, program the limbic system into seeing those behaviors as conducive to survival because we suddenly feel less threatened by our stress. Resolving modern day stress, which is not actually a threat to survival, is the missing process the Limbic System has yet to evolve. While drugs can make it go away for a while, drugs are not a viable solution, unless using more is an acceptable solution.

If we are stressed and have a beer our limbic system is conditioned that relief came from that beer and it then becomes programmed to seek the source of that relief when troubles or threatening events like stress occur. It gives us an easy out to avoid the awareness of uncomfortable thoughts and feelings instead of making healthy responses and decisions, which could actually really resolve the discomfort or stress cause. Let's look more closely at the limbic system and its intended function.

Limbic Function

The limbic system reacts with and/or controls basically three areas:

1. Food
2. Sex
3. Safety

This is why all our compulsive/addictive behaviors are in these three areas.

The Addicted Brain

Let's examine why addiction is so troublesome and hard to stop or reverse. I was attending a professional training in the late 90's when a popular relapse prevention guru named Terence Gorski briefly addressed the addicted brain in regards to the limbic system. This brief moment was a turning point for me as a professional because it identified for me a clearer understanding of why addicts use and use. He stated that events come through our senses and are fed into various parts of the brain. The limbic system labels these events with different degrees of response or severity as either safe or dangerous. If tagged dangerous because of the experience or past trauma, either real or imagined, it reacts by creating anxiety or sadness. If the event is tagged as having to do with survival, the limbic system can create a focused impulse for a specific behavior that has been associated with survival regarding this stressor in the past. In essence; what worked the last time. The inclination or craving focuses our attention on that behavior until we feel safe or normal again. If a recalled behavior is utilized again then the sought out behavior becomes more reinforced/conditioned and thereby becomes a method of coping with the perceived stressor.

An Addiction is Born

In its simplest form, addiction is not about getting high or getting a buzz, but instead it is about providing the user with a way to feel more normal, safer, free from stress and sometimes free from a sense of impending doom. The conscious mind learns to cooperate with the learned behavior (getting high when things aren't feeling good or ok) and protects this process from being challenged by a defense mechanism called denial (covered earlier during the Self-Deception discussion.) The result of this process is a brain that is emotionally or psychologically "addicted" to this favored pattern of behavior and relief.

Emotional Reactions and Limbic Deception

If the limbic system is negatively programmed during our early development by high-stress traumatic experiences it will become programmed to respond to future stressors with whatever behavior it adopted to deal with that particular stressor at that time it occurred. For example; If a child growing up in a dysfunctional family that used shouting to address conflict, developed the habit of going to their room and isolating whenever voices got loud then this individual is very likely to flee elevated voices as an adult. The behavior to avoid or escape loud tones has thus been programmed into the limbic system because it worked. As we stated in an earlier chapter, the limbic system does not have rational abilities thus it is not able to process concepts like time, or even who is doing the shouting. Therefore it (the human limbic system in this case) experiences the loud and threatening voices as if they were days apart instead of decades apart. This is especially true when there are other similarities involved like gender, tone, family role, location, and even the specific content of the shouting.

One of the reasons why substance abuse has such a strong hold over the user is that using helps a person believe they are in control of how they feel. They learn that by administering the drug they can medicate themselves to control their feelings and avoid unpredictable and uncomfortable emotions. By using a specific drug of choice they know how they will feel despite what goes on around them. They can "turn off" worry, conflict, poor self-worth, fear and stress.

This is obviously a false sense of control. Keeping this ill-lusion alive is only achieved through repeated use. These behaviors, which usually involve instant-gratification only lead to more compulsiveness which eventually evolves into full scale, full blown, substance addiction. Their addictive behaviors are only a temporary respite from their insecurities and fears. Their substance of choice only temporarily removes the awareness of the unwanted thoughts and feelings. This is Why They "must" Use, again and again.

Using a drug that makes the feelings of stress go away does not change the reality of the stressor, only the uncomfortable feelings and emotions related to it. For the addict to recover they must, in the strictest sense of the words, "change their mind." They must stop their minds from using the escape route afforded by their substance. To change their minds they must learn how to reprogram their brain by first discovering these falsehoods and erroneous beliefs. Then they must replace these falsehoods with the truth and more positive/productive behaviors, which actually resolve the stressors and not mask their existence.

Once they are detoxed and this new learning process begins, they will get brief glimpses of their false programming. They will begin to realize that they have been reinforcing these false beliefs, which in truth have actually been sabotaging their progress towards a comfortable, safe and stabile life.

The truth is that in order for this change to take place they will need to learn to trust in something greater then a drug. Their best chances to trust usually manifest in a belief in a God, or in a creation of their own Higher Power. They must also find power in other people who have overcome their struggles.

The limbic system will make it very difficult for them to make these changes because it involves risk and risks are fearfull. (Risk by definition; suggests potential loss.) There must be a safe environment for this trust to develop. It cannot happen on the family battleground or while engaged in office politics, as these scenarios are perceived as too vital for survival to the limbic system. Discord in these dynamics threatens happiness and they thereby ignite fight or flight reactions, which by extension cause cravings for the addict. They will not be successful unless it feels safe for them to let down their guard and take risks. Amends will come much later.

Issues that might bring up feelings of shame must be avoided at all costs unless in a clinical setting or a recovery program. It is rarely safe for the human animal to take risks alone. One reason why recovery programs work so well is because the people who participate often vocalize their own shortcomings and defects with reckless abandon. There is no shame in AA, NA, GA, DA or Al-Anon and Nar-Anon, only support, hope, love and encouragement. (Get some!)

Limbic Change Happens in a Delay

Even after an addict knows and comprehends the truth, has discovered their false beliefs, and uncovered the survival falsehoods, there is a time delay between what the limbic system believes and what the rational centers of the brain has now newly learned and perceived. This delay can be a process which takes anywhere from a couple of months to several years to re-sync into a positive and productive mode. Right thinking will return if they have the opportunity to challenge the false beliefs and traumatic experiences in a safe environment. But the risk must still be taken. They may experience fear and feelings of panic, but once they are able to go through these feelings without resorting to the old behavior (using) their limbic system will actually begin to see the old behavior of using as the true threat that it is. They will transition from falsehood and illusion to truth and reality.

Remember; the limbic system is the area of the brain that experiences Post Traumatic Stress Disorder (PTSD.) The resolution to PTSD is very similar to overcoming addiction. There is a reason why people who suffer from PTSD are put in support groups and why survivors of work place or school violence are treated together. Support and safety!

Once this "changing of the mind" occurs the negative reactions will be lessened by each experience related to a survival threat. It will become less and less of a reflex/desire to resort to the old behavior of using. Not gone but lessened. With support they will be able to make a good choice rather than overreacting with an unproductive and even fake "fight or flight" response solution. Old automatic habits aren't changed quickly or easily, and they are stronger when we are Hungry, Angry, Lonely or Tired (HALT). All these emotions are related to survival. The acronym, HALT is a very popular memory device used in AA to caution members against allowing their emotions to get to dangerous levels in certain key areas known to increase the alcoholic/addict's potential to relapse. As mentioned before; hunger, anger, lack of a mate (loneliness) and sleep, are all human survival needs.

Many recovering addicts and trauma survivors have programmed the survival part of their brains (Limbic System) with thousands and thousands of instances of avoiding unwanted thoughts or emotions. The amount of times they have reinforced these behaviors is staggering (no pun intended but it is interesting don't you think?) Most addicts and alcoholics cannot clearly articulate how many times they have chosen not to "fight" with their issue of addiction, but to instead take "flight" into that addiction.

Cigarette smokers reinforce their addiction hundreds of times a day by administering the drug so frequently that they can rarely estimate how many times in one day. The cigarette smoker's frequency of administration and reinforcement is why some medical professionals say nicotine addiction is harder to stop then opiate addiction. Frequency is the culprit but it is also the solution. Days without a drink, clean days, days without "ANY" cigarettes, and time away from the false beliefs are crucial for the limbic system to recover the truth.

As people repeatedly use a drug over long periods of time, this "flight" pattern becomes an automatic reaction; it becomes what most of us call a behavior or habit. Once a new identity based on new beliefs is attained they can change that "old" pattern or reprogram their limbic system to practice healthier resolutions to their discomfort. Once they get through the first year they then have a sober New Years behind them, a religious holiday, a sober 4th of July, and birthday to refer back to as a success.

You must be patient and Give Time Time, give the change a chance to happen. While the recovery process is hard for the addict, I believe it can be even more difficult for the loved ones. It is the reason I wrote this book. As a clinician I rarely find people more emotionally tortured then those persons who love an addict or alcoholic. Perhaps the most difficult thing of all is to do nothing and hope for the best.

Change happens in these areas one decision at a time, One day at a time. They can't let their "lying" emotions tell them it would feel good to do the drugs, the alcohol, the sex, or even the food. They must learn to listen to the part of their brain that has recently learned the truth and do what is truly the best or right thing, right now. If they continue to apply these new practices they will begin to break the deadly pattern of use, and decrease the time that the limbic falsehoods exist.

Oh yeah! Just one relapse, one use of the chemical will reset the process, reinforce the addiction, and remind the limbic system of their old survival deception. Each successive use further reinforces the problem. ALL USE MUST STOP FOR THIS PROCESS TO CORRECT ITSELF.

Compulsion

Because issues related to addiction are very complex and result from an intermingling of unimaginable variables, it is important to remember to keep things simple. The issues and resolutions related to compulsions are simple, not easy. One of my main hopes is to provide you with the necessary level of understanding you need, so I will not waste time trying to split hairs or speculate about cause and effect any more than we already have. I'm sure you spend enough time doing that with your addict.

A craving is in essence a desire. It is a whim, desire or want created in the human mind. Desire is not believed to be present in most other animal species, only instinct. This human construct of a "whim or desire," is related to what the human mind perceives to be enjoyable or pleasant. Not "needed" but "wanted." Most animals are not seen as having wants; they are believed to be acting out of a need for survival, instinct. This is not to say that some monkeys don't like better trees or fruits then others, but some academics argue these choices are still based on "perceived survival needs". Arguing these types of issues or facts are the "splitting hairs" I warned you about.

133

While the issue of cravings may have prehistoric origins for attaining necessary nutrients lacking in the body, the evolution of human society seems to have relegated that necessary mechanism to flights of fancy and self-gratification. What you want to eat is very different from just needing to eat.

Most social scientists are convinced that if the human body is supplied with the vital nutrients needed for survival that a craving for a specific substance becomes a short duration event, one of only about 9 seconds long.

Here is a very generalized example. Let's say you're sitting on the sofa watching TV when a craving presents itself for some chocolate. Your intra-personal communication might go something like this: "Chocolate, is there any in the house? No, darn." Either the craving for chocolate is dismissed because you are certainly not going to the store in the raging snowstorm or, you begin to contemplate how you might attain some chocolate or even who might have some nearby.

At this time the short duration craving becomes something else. What was once an emotional "whim or desire" now becomes a goal, a mental process or even an obsession to a small degree. No longer a desire, the individual is now faced with a "requirement of perception only." The object now becomes a supposed need. This is now a mental obsession and not a physical body event. The compulsion aspect of the craving has been overruled by the obsession of the mind.

Let's get back to the chocolate. We might ask ourselves: Is it worth risking my life for chocolate in this snowstorm? At this point the rational mind that has not been tainted by conditioning of disproportionate emotional reward (like substance addiction) ceases the quest for the chocolate as not being a significant enough gain in contrast to the risk to attain it. Another point that may shed some light on this dynamic is that had you been distracted by something captivating on the TV you might have forgotten all about the chocolate before you ever got past the 9 second mark. The mind moves on past the craving when other thoughts and input occupy the senses.

The addicted mind is different. The addicted mind has become convinced by conditioning to perceive the reward experienced as both valuable and necessary. The healthy mind does not see the chocolate as necessary or worth the risk. While the perceived need may be erroneous to the rational mind the emotional mind of the addict contributes immense significance and gain from the "desired" substance. The intrapersonal communication in the addicted mind might go like this. "I could be snowed in here for days and I will go crazy with no beer or weed." At this point the addict has begun to obsess about the chemical and the mind is no longer operating from a purely survival need born of the limbic system: The addicted mind is instead operating from a very convoluted mix of desire, experience/conditioning and even fear (survival). This feeling of needing the chemical is in fact a delusion, as the human body does not require these chemicals. For millions of years the human animal's survival was much more threatened then it is now. Actually, we have never had it so good when it comes to survival. We have government aid, soup kitchens, entitlement programs, police and firemen. It has actually become quite hard to die from lacking anything in the United States.

Now back to the chocolate. I know some of you are still wondering about the chocolate. No? Did you forget about it again? You were distracted. Is this book interesting enough to distract you? You have probably already moved past the idea of the chocolate, past the 9 seconds of the craving but I understand, I brought it back up. Now what is it called?

135

My reminding you of the chocolate is for a reason. Reminders batter the addicted mind, 24-7. My reminder is a lot like the majority of stimulus in the addict's world. They can barely walk down the street without being confronted by cues to use. Think about how often you might be reminded about something you might desire. Multiply that by 1000. Even if the addict can get past the cravings and the triggers for use there is always another around the corner and they can appear almost anywhere. An empty glass in the dishwasher can trigger a chronic alcoholic, and the heroin addict can be triggered by the spoon. These reminders are everywhere.

Next time you drive through a city or town or your local main thoroughfare, try counting the number of liquor stores or bars along the way. You might not see them but the alcoholic does. Now try removing the snowstorm mentioned earlier and replace the bars and liquor stores with chocolate stores. Are you stopping to get some yet? I promise your conditioning for chocolate is nowhere near as strong as the addict's desire for their drug of choice.

Multiply their brief craving, which happens 1000's of times a day, to their conditioning for the drug, to their mental obsessions for the security perceived in the substance and you might have an idea of the overwhelming task they face. Again, just another reason Why They Use and use and use.

PART VI

ENABLING

Where Do We Draw The Line?

Why do you think it is that the loved ones of an alcoholic or drug addict try to rationalize with a person who is suffering from a mental illness? Wait, did you get that? Rational and mental illness; aren't these two things mutually exclusive? Isn't that why we call it a mental illness in the first place, because it's not logical: Because it doesn't make rational sense?

If it's a person's behavior that we don't like then it is most likely a behavioral problem and not necessarily a logical or rational problem at all. As mentioned earlier the addict has become conditioned through a long process of chemical reward. Their discomfort is treated with the reward of the cessation of that discomfort via the administration of the drug.

This behavioral verses rational argument blurs an already fine line when it comes to addiction. The only way to get a person to change a behavior is to make the behavior not worth doing, by adding a sanction or penalty. This part of the brain (the limbic system) in truly the animal part of the human brain, thus there is a need to address this part of the human brain much like we would train the brain of any other animal.

As discussed in the chapter about self-deception and denial, the addict has an uncanny ability to avoid the memory of and/or retention of any information, which is contrary to their desired belief. Any information, which might threaten the justification of their use or using behaviors, is systematically eliminated from their consciousness. If a loved one is a source of stress about the issue and is continuously pushing or pursuing the issue they will eventually eliminate that loved one from their daily life. This is the reason why they appear to choose using and using friends over the people who really love them. I'll say this is again: This is the reason; "the how" they are able to choose using over the people who love them.

Take this author's word when I say; "Your contribution and worth to them is eerily irrelevant until long after they have lost you." Threats against cutting them off are only perceived as you choosing your wants over their needs. To them you are simply making things harder than they should be or need to be. They must actually "BE" cut off; threats are useless against their deep-seated denial.

The reason I say it takes the actual loss of a loved one is mostly because they will not perceive or believe the loss initially. Their using of the chemical will alleviate the very feeling of loss. Even after you have separated yourself from them they will find reasons that you are to blame for the relationship's struggles. Quitting use of the substance is rarely an option to the addict until well after great loss has occurred and then only when the user has recognized the loss. You can't spare them anything but the consequences of their use and that is enabling in its strictest sense. The addict will not stop using until the cost of using is greater than the benefits of using.

If you have an addict in your life you have obviously considered the term "Enabling" before you opened this book: But do you have a working definition? I think the definition I use will help you to clear things up and maybe even speed up the recovery of your addict.

The definition I use is as follows; **Enabling is any action by any one, that insulates or protects the substance user from the actual or potential consequences of their use.** This definition should be simple enough to understand but I urge you to take a second look at it and consider your actions in regards to your addict. Unfortunately for the significant others of the addict and alcoholic the word "Love" often becomes over simplified and trivialized. They may even use the word love as a method of instilling guilt in you, to get you to do what they want/need you to do.

I want to acknowledge here that I understand that stopping enabling behaviors is hard but I promise you it is the quickest and safest route to creating CHANGE in their behavior. At a minimum, it is a way of starting your own healing process because you can't gamble your peace of mind or make it contingent on the choices of an addict. You will come up short every time.

Popular enabling behaviors include but ARE NOT LIMITED TO: Giving them a roof over their head when they have failed to maintain their own roof due to using and poor choices. Lending them money for any reason. (Duh!) If they're hungry then feed them, never give them money. But before you feed them let them know that they will have to talk about their choices during the meal, not after. If they don't agree then they are just making another bad choice. When they are hungrier an hour later they will be learning more about their poor choices and become even more willing to have the uncomfortable discussion, mostly because the discomfort of their hunger is a stronger survival need.

Don't pay for lawyers! Jail is a consequence and not having money to pay for their own legal needs are sometimes a consequence of using as well. Being afraid is a consequence of use. <u>Let them be afraid.</u>

The only thing I suggest you might provide for them is LOW COST TREATMENT opportunities. Sending them to a "nice" place is often and can actually be counterproductive. Addiction isn't nice. If you are an addict and need treatment and can go to a nice place, then go. If you can't afford a "nice" place then act accordingly. The only adjustment to this rule is if there are other more complicated issues to address like childhood sexual abuse, trauma or major grief issues, which can be correlated to the onset of their addictive use. It's been my experience that "nice" treatment centers are usually the first treatment centers and rarely the last. But it is a process; sometimes this de-evolution in treatment quality can serve as a benchmark system for them to see their decline and to mark the progression of their illness. Again, this process would only suggest that the "nice" treatment center is only the "first" treatment center. Don't waste YOUR money!

As mentioned before the issue of addiction is extremely complicated. Rarely are the choices without controversy. This is often the case when the care of the children of the addict is in question and required. The issue will arise regarding the safety of and the care of their children. The answer to this dilemma is more straightforward then you might expect. By taking care of the children you are not aiding the addict per say, you are aiding innocent victims of a disease state. This is not enabling. The children deserve the best we can afford for them or they too will be visited by many of the addict's troublesome emotional states and behaviors.

This does not mean that the addict has to be granted visitation with the children. Where the issues of consequence and enabling really get confusing is when it comes to their visitation and whether or not the addicted person should be able to see their children while they are still using. This is often a complicated dynamic but if the rules are in place ahead of time the path can be smoother. I could write an entire book on this subject, as the issue is important. Children need stability and predictability, rarely traits attributed to a practicing addict.

Quite simply visitation should happen at times arranged by the new caregiver and at a time when the caregiver and the child are not inconvenienced. This is mostly because the using person will often not show up for the arranged time. Their inability to make these important connections with "their" children can be a significant consequence when they are confronted by the reality of a missed opportunity. I recommend establishing a 15 minutes rule. No more than 15 minutes early and no more than 15 minutes late. No excuses should be entertained, as we all know, when something is important enough we are on time and prepared for that event.

Now I can already hear the voices saying; what about the children? They need to see their parents. Well, kind of, no they don't. Not addicted, unkempt, emotionally unstable ones. This can be an important life lesson for the child when the addict falls short. Addiction causes hurt, pain and missed opportunity.

Just as you need to do for yourself, you have to aid the child in depersonalizing the addict's failure to comply. When possible I recommend that the child not be told of arranged meeting times because they will, more times than not, not show. Children are not tools or apparatuses used to instill change in an addict. You may be faced with the issue of peace orders or restraining orders. Better safe than sorry. An estranged person who violates such an order may find the clarity that only this situation can provide. They must experience the results of their choices, and feel their own consequences.

One of the most flagrant of all possible enabling misdeeds you might commit to another significant other, is the neglecting and wasting of resources (time, money, love). Don't deny the children something because you are using that money to "help" the addicted. I have seen countless examples of difficulties resulting from over focus on the addicted. Want to improve the family as a whole? De-emphasize the addict in daily life. Don't let them consume you and your resources with their overwhelming sense of urgency and self-pity. Let them learn that their choices cause their consequences.

Now this might be a little confusing at first. With all that in mind I want you to remember to reward the positive actions. We might call it "abling." If you see the addict making positive steps try reinforcing the positive behavior by arranging a sort of bonus meeting. Maybe you put together an impromptu meeting or quick meal at a favorite fast food place of the child. For instance; Bobby and I were going to John Doe's burger joint and wanted to know if you wanted to join us there.

I know it's hard to grasp sometimes but the truth is that love by way of support doesn't correlate to addicts getting into recovery. Only perceived loss, strong boundaries, limitations and consequences will push them to acceptance, to the reality of their unmanageability, their disease and by extension their need for recovery. NEVER REWARD THE BEHAVIOR AHEAD OF TIME

Finally, have you ever known anyone who was in major denial about something besides addiction? When did the denial end? It ended when the truth could no longer be denied or avoided. Enabling helps the addict deny the reality of the

142

situation and prolongs their awareness of the truth. Addicts use because they can still use and meet their other needs like food, clothing, shelter and staying out of jail. The problem with you helping is that they will never come to believe that your assistance will ever stop unless it stops. One reason they believe they can still use is because they see you and other enablers as their failsafe. You need to let them know that they have used up and exhausted that failsafe.

Once addicted the flood gates are open and they can't be closed until the flood is over. I once heard it said that; "Using drugs is like making love to a gorilla. Once you start, you aren't done till the gorilla's done." Addiction is only done when it has used up everyone around the addict and everything inside the addict. Long-term recovery will not occur until this has happened. Consequences are sometimes seen as a method of raising the bottom for the substance abuser.

Why They Use and Use?

The Big Let Down or a Reversal of Effect

Nearly everyone who has ever administered a mood altering substance to his or her body has done so for an effect. Even those persons who sought to gain social standing by going with the group (peer pressure) used the drug for an effect. Thus everyone who administers a mood-altering drug wants to change something about his or her current emotional state otherwise there would be no need for the use of a mood-altering drug. One might argue that at some level the user is not currently content with the way s/he feels and that the individual wants to feel different.

Even those persons, who consider themselves happy and well adjusted, understand that the chemical will have an effect, desired or not. Any person knowing that the chemical being administered has mood altering effects must therefore be seeking to alter their conscious condition. Do not be fooled. What this means is that they are not 100% satisfied with their current state of mind as they are seeking to better it, improve it or heighten it. Even using a caffeinated beverage meets these criteria of desiring to change ones' current mood or state.

With this in mind let's narrow our focus to further examine how the addict becomes this way. If it is true that the addicted person began their using to medicate a state of mind that they were not content with then the path is much clearer. After a while the emotional fog of substance use takes over in the addict and the lines between "me" and "me altered" become blurred. The altered mood becomes so familiar to the user that they get fooled into thinking that the way they are under the influence of the chemical is their natural condition; "me altered" becomes "me" (and me un-altered becomes an uncomfortable state.)

Over the past twenty-five years I have met with more substance abusers and substance dependents then I can count. When they are asked; "Why they use?" Nearly all, (99.9%) struggle to provide a coherent response to which they themselves are satisfied. Nearly all have failed to articulate a substantial rationale for a behavior that by this time has cost them; jobs, relationships, freedom, self-respect and even their health. The few who can answer to their own satisfaction say, "Because I don't care anymore."

Getting to a point where they are satisfied with their answer has frequently required a fair amount of facilitation to help them articulate and arrive at a cohesive understanding of the using behavior. Sometimes the full awareness of their motivation can take months and even years to uncover. While answers like, "because I like it," are often suggested these fail to explain the gain or motive for the costly behavior. What this suggests to me is that outside of their emotional addiction/habit, no existing cognitive reason is actually present. This most likely occurs because the original reason or motive to use has become long lost in the disease process of addiction.

While this may sound a little absurd, it is no less true. Remember, it's a mental illness not a rational process. The reason is quite simply that the original impetus for use has changed without their knowing it. The addict now uses to feed the emotional illness and their physiological addiction (treating withdrawal). They no longer gain or experience the original benefit of the behavior.

Let's examine this further. I go grocery shopping for a reason, I go to work for a reason, I have a wife/lover for a reason. Our actions are motivated by our needs, drives, desires and sometimes by what other people ask of us (doing it for others still contains a motive). The addict doesn't really have a motive outside of feeling better right now. It's usually (90% of the time) about treating their withdrawal. When the addicted use, what they are truly seeking is to "not" feel what they feel when the effect of the drug is gone. They are not using to feel good. What they are doing is using to not feel "bad." Reality is too uncomfortable, and they respond with statements like; "I don't know who I am without it" and "not having it makes me uncomfortable."

One point that I hope you take from this chapter and this book as a whole is that addiction is not a behavior born of rational choice. Addicts use because their brains have become hi-jacked by a disease that is spiritual, mental/emotional and physical. They have become "erroneously" convinced through conditioning and the fear of discomfort, that the only way to escape their discomfort is to have access to their drug of choice.

Loved ones of the user/addict often suffer with the user's choices believing that their behavior takes place while conscious of the consequences and of the affect it will have on others. I promise you it does not. The same "dope fiend" that will steal his grandmother's medication will become appalled at the mention of the act when in their "right mind." A toxic mind cannot be of right mind. As a person who loves them you cannot try to account for your own worth and value based on the addict's behavior or choice. I KNOW YOU DO!

Addicts are often seen as some of the most selfish people in society. Addicts are people who can't do the "right" thing for themselves. What they have become is self-absorbed. If they can't do it for themselves then how can they do it for anyone else? The addict is not necessarily self-ish. That term selfish suggests a slighter degree of self-ish-ness, as sort of being overly self-centered. The addict lives at such an intense level of fear and discomfort that they have to become self-absorbed. It's not about the "self," not really. The idea of a "self" is a fairly long gone phenomenon by this point. The chemical is first and foremost. The chemical makes more of the choices then the addict and chemicals are NOT RATIONAL.

Developmental Exposure

As discussed in some of the earlier chapters on the "Models of Addiction Treatment" many of the treatment approaches developed over the past 100 years suggested that addiction might actually be born in a child's early developmental process. My foremost suggestion here is for you to remember that it is impossible to reverse history. Regardless of the initial factors that lead to addictive use the problem of motivation to use shifts during the addictive process of the disease. Oncologists don't spend much time figuring out what caused someone to have lymphoma. They confirm the state then move forward with a resolution. The time they would waste trying to determine why a person got cancer would only slow down the onset of treatment. Just like in cancer treatment, this may be something to try to determine after the important or more vital phases of treatment have been completed.

It won't be long before we have a genetic test to determine if someone might be more at risk of becoming an addict but we still won't be able to guess which children will. All children face some kind of dysfunction in their childhood and only a relatively small percentage become addicted.

PLEASE: Wasting your time second-guessing yourself or the parents of a loved one is ridiculous in regards to dealing with the addict or treating the illness. It is about as useful as knowing who gave you a cold. While it does seem to be a part of human nature to place blame, blame doesn't resolve a single thing whether it's you blaming yourself or someone else. You will need all the help and energy you can muster to deal with this problem. Don't let them distract you by suggesting their addiction was someone else's doing! The addicted will use history in an attempt to defocus from the problem at hand. They are lost in false rationale. They are not rational human beings while they are addicted and probably not for a substantial period of time after they stop using. Their best thinking has failed them.

Socialization of Addiction

Much like the above discussion suggested it is often a knee-jerk reaction to place blame. While the initial cause of the problem may be irrelevant to the treatment of the problem there are real social and environmental causes for continued use and relapse. Once again, certain factors may influence individual choices but since not all people who are exposed to those same influences make the same choices, placing the blame in those areas must be suspect.

Growing up in a family that owns a bar does not make you an alcoholic. Growing up with addicted parents does not make you a drug addict. Growing up with a father who is a serial killer does not make you a murderer. At some level, at some time, and at some place a personal choice is made; an experience is had and then another choice is made. Each personal choice made diminishes the correlation between the environmental influence and the outcome. It is also important to remember that one choice and one event does not make one an addict.

So how many poor choices does it take? There is an old saying; "when you're in a hole, stop digging." When you find yourself in a house on fire, get out! The number of poor choices is not as germane to success as the specific situations and options. Options allow a person to seek alternatives to negative choices. We provide options through educating and communicating. Does a child have an option between just hanging out on a street corner or playing ball? If we don't provide the option then we have failed.

Before we begin arguing all the semantics let's remember that what caused the problem is not so much the point of this book. We are trying to understand; *"Why They Use."* Yes, environmental issues can lead to use but many people in those same environments do not become addicted, so cause and effect must still be questioned. Many people use without becoming addicted. Lots of people abuse substances but do not become dependent.

I would like to improve your clarity on how socialization issues can lead to relapse. The factors here are quite simple; Using peers, special occasions, holidays, paydays, stress, weddings, funerals, etc... Layer some of these factors together and the addict is easily overwhelmed. Addicts who don't verbally confess their "now clean and sober status" to their communities are much more likely to be offered drugs and alcohol. (Not disclosing the status suggests there are reservations in their acceptance of powerlessness, which suggests they don't really want to change.) The people who know the addict have a preconceived notion of their propensity to use and are, more times than not, only being social when they offer a habitual user a substance. Until these disclosures are made the addict's recovery is in grave danger. The first step of any 12-step program is admission and honesty, as in We admitted we were powerless over ... -that our lives had become unmanageable.

Conditioning

One of the causal factors often suggested in an attempt to make sense of the irrational behavior of substance addiction and relapse is believed to be the result of "conditioning." However, as mentioned earlier in the paradigm on "The Behavioral Model of Addiction," human conditioning is the product of repetition not exposure. A single event may become a fond memory but it is not conditioning. Repeating the positive experience of an earlier event successfully is what leads to conditioning.

Hopefully this scenario will help make my point. If I go over to your house for dinner and I experience the best meal of my life then I have a very fond memory of the event. I may even try to get myself invited back for more of what I experienced. At this point all we really have is knowledge of a positive experience centered on the good food you served (recall the limbic system and how its relation to food is survival oriented and not a rational process.) If upon my return to your wonderful kitchen the experience is only "so-so," then I chalk it up to something different, a fluke maybe. Should you recreate the first experience for me or even out do yourself then I am on my way to becoming conditioned to believe that you ='s good food. There may even come a time, after several blissful experiences that my mouth begins to water when I hear your name or see you on my caller ID. (Just like Pavlov's Dog.)

Now let's imagine that there is an outside environmental or social factor that occurs while I'm there. Say the diner is great but your dog bites me. Now the moment of choice comes when I am invited back. I will have to determine the "risk" verses "reward" scenario. If I knowingly return after being invited back to your house and your dog bites me again I have a role in this decision, I have still made a choice despite your dog's temperament, to re-experience the reward of your cooking. In much this same way the addict is willing to be bitten in order to re-experience the moments of bliss.

The above process is very similar to the addicts experience with their drug of choice; it's exactly what happens to a person who chooses to experiment with mood altering substances. The person has a reaction to the experience of use that can range from very negative to blissful. The determining factor in whether it is a good or bad experience is usually related to the mindset of the individual at the time of use (Mind set being everything from self-worth to physical health.) Because socialization and environment help to predetermine the mindset of the individual using the substance, the substance itself is not initially seen as inherently bad (like your dog). That is why we say drugs have a potential for addiction and dependency, graded from low to high. Conditioning occurs either slowly or quickly depending on the frequency of use, the chemical used, the duration between use experiences, and the emotional state of the person taking the substance.

Most people refer to someone who does something a lot as an addict. He's addicted to tv, to video games, she's a chocoholic, an exercise junkie, a shop-aholic, workaholic, etc... While repeated use can become a habit and part of a routine it does not qualify as "addiction" per say. The person may be "overdoing it" but this is not the same as chemical or substance addiction. For the purposes of this book we will focus only on the issue at hand, substance addiction and *Why They Use*. When focusing on addiction, unmanageability and loss of control related to use is what determines abuse; tolerance and withdrawal determine dependency. Physical dependence is usually diagnosed as a condition that presents when a particular substance is removed from the physical body and a state of withdrawal (shock) develops.

While a young lady's heavy use of chocolate and sudden cessation of use may create the withdrawal symptom of a headache it is because of the addiction to the caffeine in the chocolate and not the chocolate. Beer drinkers aren't addicted to the taste of the beer they are addicted to the alcohol in the beer and the cessation of the alcohol causes the physiological reaction.

What Dr. Pavlov (discussed earlier) determined was that the animal brain quickly begins to associate stimuli with perceived gain without conscious thought being applied. This adaptation in behavior is a natural response to perceived gain. Let's be clear that "perceived gain" is a crucial element here. The gain only has to be perceived, it does not have to be real. Pavlov eventually stopped feeding the dog after the bell. The dog still salivated without the actual reward of food. He continued to do so until the conditioned response (drooling) was extinguished.

The addict's problem is that s/he has been deeply and thoroughly conditioned. The longer and more intense the use the longer the extinguishing takes. This extinction process needs to be consistent as "using again" even just once completely re-ignites the addicted's emotional connection or conditioned response. This is why abstinence is the only solution for the substance dependent person. Each use of any mood altering substance threatens to return the user to the prior state of irrational emotional connection to their substance of choice. I have also written a book for the addicted as well called Addiction: Am I Powerless (Self Assessing, A user's guide to the truth). (Addictioninthefamily.com)

Emotional Dependence

Have you ever depended on someone for something? Did it work out for you? Aren't there people we believe we could not live without or if we were to lose them, doesn't it seem like life just wouldn't be the same, wouldn't be as enjoyable? Of course! Well the addict has an emotional dependence on their substance in much the same way. When everyone else in their world makes them feel bad the drug always helps, always does what its "supposed" to do. If nothing else it is reliable. Thus an emotional dependence is formed in much the same way a dependence on people is, through experience (positive reinforcement.)

Most addicts have two different states of dependency existing within them at the same time. One state is an emotional dependency and the other state is a physical dependency. We'll discuss the emotional dependency first. As we have discussed in earlier chapters the addict has often falsely programmed their brains to believe that the world and its people have let them down; that they are the victims of a lack of insight and understanding by others. They have also programmed their brains to believe that the chemical they use is a solution to their problems. The experiences of using the chemical and getting relief from their stress falsely convinces them that it is helping them to survive and it thus becomes an indispensable part of their being "OK." This is an emotional dependence.

When diagnosing addiction we use the earlier described variances of either Substance Abuse or Substance Dependence. When diagnosing the condition of Substance Dependence we first establish the presence of the Substance Abuse Criteria and then add to it the diagnosed presence/existence of tolerance and/or withdrawal.

154

Withdrawal is diagnosed by the pathological condition that presents when a particular substance is removed from the physical body and a physical reaction develops or occurs. This is a type of shock to the system created by the absence of the chemical the body has now adjusted to having present. This is physiological dependence.

PART VII

Stumbling Blocks to Stepping Stones

Fear/Anger

"Driven by a hundred forms of fear, self delusion, self seeking and self pity we steps on the toes of our fellows and they retaliate." This line is from page 62 of the book "Alcoholics Anonymous" in the chapter titled "How It Works." Is it any wonder, Why They Use? What are these hundred forms of Fear?

The addict's greatest fear is quite simply that they will not have enough. Their fear is that they will not have enough of anything and everything; but mostly that they will not have enough of the substance needed; the one that makes everything else, OK. The addict's second biggest fear and a great cause of an addict's anxiety is that someone or something will get in the way of, or in between them and their substance. Think about that for just a second. Their second biggest fear is often our first approach to the problem. "STOP USING!" we shout at them, you need to stop right now. What we are actually doing is forcing them to choose, usually on the spot, between us and their best friend and love of their life. We have thus created one of the primary states that they have conditioned themselves to treat with the drug. We create more stress and more anxiety and even more cravings.

Recall from the earlier chapter on the limbic system when we discussed "fight or flight." Remember that the original stress of mankind and other animals was to survive. Remember that the addict has been falsely conditioned to believe that their drug is vital to survival, that it saves them from threats. When we threaten the drug we threaten a CORE survival response in the addict who has a type of false or faulty programming. It might be like clicking on your Internet Explorer tab and having Word open. Once the link is clicked it's going to open Word. In order to fix that "erroneous programming" you are going to have to reprogram that part of the operating system. Much like the computer their faulty programming will have them half way down the street with no way to reverse the process. Before they realize that the wrong program has initiated they will have fled the scene. After their limbic response has dissipated they realize they've been running from and feeling threatened by their grandmother.

Following these primary fears based in the limbic system, the spectrum of fear gets even more broad. Half the fears that present evolve into numerous types and varying displays of anger. An old AA program saying supported by many psychotherapists suggests; "Anger is fear turned inside out" that there are only two major emotions; Love and Fear, and that all other emotions and "character traits" arise from those two base emotions. Clinically this is not far from the truth with most psychotherapists being in concert that most negative emotions do indeed arise from fear. This is also true of neurosis based mental health issues like anxiety, panic, phobias, and self esteem issues; they are all based in fear. In regards to Limbic system based responses, anger is simply a leaning towards the "fight side" of the fight or flight response.

Until the alcoholic/addict accepts the premise that their substance is merely a symptom of their problem their hopes for recovery are short lived at best. When this belief fades they often return to use. While they might achieve some measure of stability and time away from the drink or drug they must resolve the issue of their faulty programming or they will use again. It is important to remember that whether or not a mental health issue existed before their substance abuse and dependency, that Substance Abuse and Substance Dependency are mental health conditions in and of themselves. In fact, Addiction is one of the deadliest of mental health conditions. That condition must be treated. Simply taking away the substance is no more treatment for the addict then telling the agoraphobic to stay home. If you want a weed to stop growing you must take out the root. Until the addict accepts responsibility and takes an honest inventory of them selves' change is almost always short lived. This self assessment/inventory process is the core of all 12-step programs.

Using reinforces its self every time it occurs. Relapse is a reinforcement of their prior conditioning, because they will "feel better" initially. Addiction is a conditioned response for both the physical body and psyche; physically, because it often halts the discomfort of withdrawal and psychologically because it provides the user with an emotional resolution to their stress-full (cognitive) discomfort. For the addict a major cause of cognitive duress or discomfort results from not allowing "sense" to make sense. When issues can't be rationally figured out, the human brain resorts back to a defensive posture as the anxiety turns into a sense of impending doom.

While psychosis is often viewed as a departure or separation from truth and reality, neurosis is the refusal to truly accept what one knows as the truth. Addiction is a mental illness that sometimes presents with both neurotic and psychotic symptoms often creating fear levels in the addict/alcoholic that are overwhelming.

Gender and Using

While addiction is a medical condition, a disease, the resulting complications of the disease can vary greatly with gender. These variances between how addiction affects men and women may result from obvious differences in physical make-up, but also include substantial differences in socialization during both childhood and adult experiences. While it can be argued that metabolism and hormone differences affect the nature of the disease the majority of the gender differences seem to be more related to issues of socialization and programming. An entire book could be written to discuss this issue so I will focus only briefly on this subject in regards to relapse potential.

Because this is not a book about the physiological aspects of the disease and physical gender differences, I'll leave those discussions to the medical professionals and biologists. However, when considering the obvious differences it should be noted that outside of physical segregation to avoid sexual contact, the majority of treatment programs in this country make little if any adjustment for physical and socialization differences in their treatment programs and treatment protocols.

Male Issues

One of the most identified emotional struggles for men regarding addiction is the popularly held belief that men are more reluctant to share their emotional vulnerability and that they are less likely to talk about their needs or desires. We'll jump right in by stopping for a moment to reflect on the issue of "talking about their needs or desires." Please note that as we have already discussed in great detail, that the major reason addicts keep using is that they have become convinced that they "NEED" the drug. This should already identify for you a major problem in the attainment of clean time for men. If I'm a man

160

and I don't talk about my "needs" and on top of that I am fearful that you will interfere with my needed substance then you can see we are at an impasse and a serious obstacle to recovery has already presented itself. "I don't want to talk about it."

While this male impediment of discussing emotional needs has decreased some in the past several decades, the vast majority of addicts left untreated are those in the forty and over group who grew up in the John Wayne error of "big boys don't cry" and "taking your licks like a man." An addict can only "suck it up" for so long. You can't "walk-off" addiction, it's a disease, and it only gets worse.

While issues related to not being able to handle your liquor and manage your emotions, may be perceived by many adult males as a sign of weakness these signs are less obvious when you surround yourself with other males of similar dysfunction. There is a 12 Step program saying which suggest that addicts are always "seeking lower companionship." Three homeless alcoholic men sitting on the curb in the urine soaked clothing will still elevate themselves above their peers. This may be partially because of the innate competitiveness in men but it is usually more correlated to issues of poor self-esteem.

Another one of the obstacles to men getting sober is their inability to talk to and meet relationship prospects when clean and sober (also a self-esteem issue.) They are often confounded by the notion of approaching a woman without some liquid courage. These are social skills that many of them have never developed because their socialization and meeting women evolved out of a party or bar environment. The skill set of meeting and getting to know women sober is a difficult one for most males to acquire. If they are unsuccessful at overcoming this obstacle they are at high risk for eventual relapse as sexual encounters are often seen as their last vice.

Female Issues

Probably one of the most glaring facts about women addicts and relapse is simply this; the more attractive they are the more likely relapse is to occur. While this statement may seem controversial at first blush it is really quite simple to understand. Interested parties (men and women,) both addicted themselves or not, are more likely to enable a woman and tolerate her addictive behaviors simply because she is attractive. More attractive women are more likely to be offered a free drink in a bar or offered to share in a drug without a "monetary" exchange.

Men often enable women as a whole group, because men are willing to put up with the negative behaviors and attitudes associated with an addiction in women in order to have them as their sexual partners: This phenomena results in women going further down the scale of unmanageability and of severity, regardless of their addiction type. They are enabled. One reason is because the major potential point of confrontation in their life (their significant other) is actually supportive of their continued use. The severity of the eventual consequences increases because they are not facing the earlier more subtle consequences or warning signs of their behaviors.

It should also be mentioned that the social pressures for return to use by male partners is extreme because most men believe that women "under the influence" are more likely to engage in sex acts they would not engage in while clean and sober. This ultimately results in women struggling to grasp the true level of their powerlessness over their substance. Further, the shame related to participating in these acts while under the influence often results in more shame and guilt which overwhelms the untreated substance abuser thereby resulting in their seeking of a drug to escape their self loathing, regret and remorse. A vicious cycle for sure.

Often women become so entrenched in these behaviors that they fail to recognize that they are actually participating in a form of prostitution: Sex for drugs. Once realized, that behavior can actually evolve into prostitution for cash as the shame of having already crossed the moral line that once existed, is negated. Because of the fallacious belief that their drug is necessary for immediate survival the long-term moral belief is circumvented or rationalized away. A good treatment program will address these issues, many don't!

Addiction and the Court System

I once had a client in an alternative sentencing program ask me: "If addiction is a disease and I have it, why are they trying to put me in jail for having it?" My response was quite simple, I asked: The first time you got a DWI what happened in court? He replied: "They gave me probation" (and I reminded him that he was instructed to stop drinking and to get some help, and to get into a program). Did you stop? "Obviously not" he said. I then asked: What happened with your second DWI? "They found me guilty, put me on probation and ordered me to treatment." What happened this last (3rd) time? "They sentenced me to a year in here."

I then asked him to follow along as I explained to him what seems to be the justice system's approach to addiction and mental illness. The first time you were arrested they told you that you had a problem. The second time you were arrested they "made" you get the help that was identified in the first sentencing, which you failed to heed. This time they put you in jail not because you have a disease but for not taking responsibility to treat a condition that you now knew that you had based on your testimony at court (Remember agreeing to probation is a type of commitment to address the problem, an admission.) They sentenced you for continuing to use after being given fair warning that you would be held accountable. You were jailed for not heeding the warning, for not changing the behavior. While mental illness is a medical condition and even a legal defense, mentally ill people still have to take their meds or they will eventually be jailed for their illegal behaviors.

I think that it is important to note at this point that there are many people who work within the justice system that genuinely care about the law and seek the "right" outcome for all concerned. The justice system struggles in treating the mentally ill because they are forced to balance the consideration of the offender's mental status at the time of their crime, with trying to determine how to best protect society from being repeatedly victimized.

As animals we humans can be conditioned just like Pavlov's dog. Once again, the addict will only stop using when the perceived costs of using out weights the perceived benefits of using. All people are resistant to change until they learn the actual benefit of any proposed change. There is a reason that we stay right of the double yellow line down the middle of the street, because head on collisions hurt and cost lots of money. The perceived cost is greater than a perceived benefit. Seat belt laws are another example. Many of us only started wearing them because we did not want the fine we were told would be levied if we were caught. We did not do it because we thought it necessary, or because we needed to for health reasons, only to prevent the fine. Eventually we realized the benefit of the changed behavior.

In contrast; at the turn of the century prison meant laboring in the hot sun under miserable conditions. People were afraid to go to jail. People were given longer sentences in the past and prisoners had fewer creature comforts. If you were locked up for a drinking related crime you got the same treatment as a murderer or rapist, hard labor. Drug courts and jail house rehabilitation services have only become a part of the justice system as a means of reducing the costs of housing criminals and to take care of the systems primary responsibility of protecting society by actually addressing a problem.

Courts and Accountability

Addicts (and other mentally ill) must be held accountable for "not" treating their disease but only after certain tests are proved.

a) Did the person have adequate knowledge of their condition?
b) Was a solution (treatment) available to them?
c) Did they have the functional ability to understand their need for treatment?

The court system frequently refers to this accountability state as "criminally responsible" but this may be a misnomer. This term may be better understood by the layman's perspective of "criminally punishable." The question arises; will putting this person in prison attain our primary goals of protecting society? Is it necessary?

Only after these primary objectives are met does the rehabilitating of the offender come into question. A judge can often be heard asking the defense counsel; "what guarantee do I have that this defendant won't offend again?"

Over the past decade or so the term rehabilitation has fallen from public focus. In the mid 80's to early 90's attention was frequently drawn to the distinction between rehabilitation and "habilitation." The prefix "re" means to do again. Obviously if the function level was never attained in the first place a person can't be literally rehabilitated but will instead need to be given the tools for the first time or habilitated. This "habilitation" is our society's responsibility but primarily it is a parental responsibility to lobby public health officials for these services and to see that this type of information is available within the educational system and then thoroughly disseminated.

After several years of testifying as an expert witness I began to question whether or not I should remain in the courtroom for the verdict. While the justice system's figureheads are dedicated individuals they are not mental health professionals and 20 minutes of testimony by a professional cannot bestow upon them the knowledge necessary to resolve or treat a mental health condition. Twenty years in jail will not cure a Bi-Polar condition thus the judge is reduced to the aforementioned primary goal of protecting society. This usually means placing a mentally ill person into the regular prison system because the mental health facilities for criminals are very over burdened.

Keeping the above in mind, years of working in the addiction field did gift me with one very valuable tool. That tool was to learn how to use the system for a client's own good. As a clinical professional working with an individual client, society at large is not "my" concern. My concern is what is in the best welfare of the client in front of me and how can I get him or her to the level of understanding that gives them the needed perspective to see where their actions or inactions will lead them. My task at that time is to take advantage of the motivational forces at work in the client's life at that time. This motivational force is the threat of incarceration, the actual consequence of their behavior.

I need to use the client's fear to motivate them to get the awareness they need, via their need to pass urine tests for the courts (staying clean and sober,) attending treatment when directed, getting the education and insight available and then moving them into more positive functioning (getting a job and keeping it, etc...)

So what's the answer? We need to have sentencing suggestions for the mentally ill being determined by individuals with a certified knowledge of the human psyche and mental illness. (As I suggest this you can hear the distant screaming of the judiciary.) The people making these decisions have to be capable of determining if the individual is capable of change and/or what it will take to achieve this change for the better. At this point in time no one truly cares about what is best. Judges and prosecutors are merely playing a numbers game based on the theory of "willful misconduct" without the knowledge of how the mentally ill are controlled by their addictive disease. Addiction truly is a matter of diminished capacity.

For example; a cocaine addict who hasn't eaten for a week or slept for 5 days commits a crime of armed robbery where someone is injured. The sentence is usually around 20 years to life. Disregarding the drug's influence on this crime and the societal stigma of addiction we are left with primarily physiological factors, which all humans have experienced.

Imagine not eating for a day. How would you feel? Two? Three? Eventually survival mechanisms in the brain (the limbic system fight or flight) kick in and override rationality. At this point it is not the actual drug that causes the act of violence it is an intersect between other dynamics of sleep deprivation, malnutrition and diminished mental capacity. In most cases, once clean and sober the same individual would never consider such an act. Prison can't change a person who isn't "that way" anyway. Any parent would steal to feed their child. History has shown that in similar cases humans even resort to cannibalism.

That's just about the nutrition and the need for food; now let's examine sleep. Say you were up all night and still had to work the next day. Would it be hard? Would you be 100%? Could you drive your car the same way after 2 or 3 days without sleep as you could on any typical day? How would your temper be? Calm and easy going or would you become more irritable and reactive? The answer to all of the proceeding questions is quite obvious; you'd be diminished at best.

This is not to say that some people don't need to be incarcerated. While many people will eventually concede to having a problem some people do not have the capacity to be honest with themselves about the reality of their problem. Some of the mentally ill are so sick that change is not possible because "effective" drugs have not been created for their conditions. One reason is that the drug companies simply don't have enough demand to cover the research and regulation costs because they don't have enough customers to purchase the needed drug in order to recoup their investment. There is no money in discovering these medications.

Before we move on I want you to stop for second to consider the legal systems test for responsibility from above, and apply it to your loved one and your own decision to penalize them with a consequence for their behavior.

- Did they have adequate knowledge of the rule or boundary?
- Was a solution (treatment or alternative) available to them?
- Did they have the functional ability to understand?

Emotional Stumbling Blocks for the Addicted

Before closing I would like to leave you with a few more insights gained and validated by both my own personal clinical experience as well as the personal experiences of millions of 12 Step program members. I refer to this group as "R.-J.E.F.F." (Resentment, Jealousy, Envy, Frustration and Fear.) These 5 emotional stumbling blocks were first articulated by the author of the book Alcoholics Anonymous, William Griffith Wilson, as the primary offenders leading to a return to use (relapse.)

Resentment

This is by no means the first time we have addressed the issue of resentment in this book. Its impact cannot be given too much attention and should never be under estimated when it comes to its morbid role for the addicted.

When the word resentment is broken down we get; "*Re*" to do again/repeat, and "*Sentīre*" to feel, in essence to "feel again." Re-feeling old hurts creates emotional pain for the holder of the resentment by intensifying a negative experience and re-administering the hurt which has now been magnified by that review, resulting in a more painful victim centered memory.

In Al-Anon they say; "detach with love." However, when loved ones try to detach and move away from the addictive behaviors of the addict, the addict will retaliate by distancing himself or herself, brooding, becoming angry and then resentful. This process is unavoidable and there is no stopping it. The addict must get over their resentments on their own, "they must or it kills them."

As loved ones distance themselves from the addict the emotional moving away creates a sense of abandonment, which is a major source of addict resentment. There is a twisted core belief on the behalf of the addicted that they can create discomfort (return it) in/to the people around them by the withholding of emotional and physical contact (I know you've felt this). Their resentments propel them to purposely make you worry about where and how they are because they know that this is one of the most painful experiences you have in regards to the problem. This behavior is a manifestation of their resentment, which also now further separates them from the truth and from loving support. There is a program saying that goes; "Your disease is trying to get you alone to kill you," resentment is the mechanism at work.

While the emotional withholding is not an exclusive behavior of the addicted and persons from addicted families, this type of dysfunction is the corner stone of their relationship struggles. Many dysfunctional people operate from the perspective that by not approving of someone they somehow affect that person's future happiness. Unfortunately a paradox does present, as the moving away, is your only way, to find any peace and emotional equilibrium. Once you move away (emotionally distance yourself) they will have no way to manipulate you. Once you get over and adapt to their distancing, your emotional healing can begin. You can trust in the fact that they will keep their resentments until they pay too greatly for them and then, hopefully, let them go themselves. Remember also that every time they use they get a break from any painful emotions or dysfunction so their using will allow them to outlast you.

Resentment is probably the most emotionally infectious part of the disease of addiction with shame a very close second. The disappointment and fear that the disease manifests results in hurt feelings, emotional pain and the loss of the trust of loved ones. As mentioned above the addict only feels the pain for a

171

short time because they quickly medicate any negative feelings away. More often than not the addict will medicate until the memories of any unpleasant exchange is completely forgotten. (Ever ask them: "Don't you see what you're doing?") The fact that the user doesn't remember the pain they caused, results in even greater pain for their significant other/s, which will only evolve into more resentments in their loved one.

Jealousy & Envy

As the addicted continue to seek reasons for their pain (other than their chemical of choice or their own behaviors) their search is forced outward to the world around them. Jealousy and Envy are very close cousins but I found it easiest to remember them in this way: Envy is between two people and Jealousy is between 3 or more. A person can envy you for your nice car but is jealous of you and your attractive partner or your friendship with their friend.

Stop for a second and consider for yourself how these issues of comparison might trip up the recovering addict. Did you stop and think?

Left unchecked the two emotional reactions known as Envy and Jealousy create a sense of self-pity for the host. The problem with envy and jealousy for the addicted is that it gets them feeling sorrier for themselves then they can handle. If we are referring to the alcoholic who is already depressed because he is abusing a depressant drug then the self-pity problem is exponentially increased. As a society we are already too steeped in a victim mentality. There is no doubt that an addict steeped in self-pity will eventually use. There is a program saying; "Poor Me, Poor Me, Pour me a Drink." Once they give up hope and project themselves as a victim in any sense they will use. Mix that with the shame of addiction and their chances against measuring up to others becomes all too overwhelming for them.

One major stumbling block for their Jealousy and Envy is very simplistic and easy for all to understand; they can't use and others "get to." This hazard results when they either see or hear about others using and having a good time doing so. They instantly become Envious that their friend got high and they get Jealous that their old friends are still going out to party without them. When the addicted become wrought with both Jealousy and Envy it is time for a meeting.

Further, as you become the gatekeeper for the addicts needs being met you also become the person with whom they associate their victimization. Try not to fall into the trap. The 12 step programs have a great saying for that too. They repeat it to the newcomer when they are down and I suggest you consider it too. "It doesn't have to be this way anymore, you don't ever have to feel this bad again." Go to a meeting and find out how.

Frustration

Everyone feels frustrations and in today's world. We are all experiencing a reduction in what is often referred to as a "frustration tolerance." When emotions like frustration are experienced regularly our capacity to handle them becomes reduced as we become more irritable and more tired from the experience. It can be accurately stated that many addictions result from and are complicated by personal frustrations. Frustration hastens the addictive process as the addict attempts to treat this particular emotional state with a chemical that works great, initially.

Relapse related to decreased frustration tolerance in the addict is a problem for the simplest of all reasons: The

173

addicted's central nervous system is in layman's terms, quite simply a mess. It is akin to an electronic device that has experienced a lightning strike, circuit boards are fried, wires are melted together and "capacitors" are burnt out. The addicted have very "faulty wiring" resulting in a decreased ability to cope with this very common emotion. Complicate that by having neglected to develop important life skills and you can imagine how easily they become overwhelmed.

Unfortunately we can't simply replace the wiring or the component damaged from the lightning strike. Instead we must aid them in overcoming the deficits that present after the damage is done by the proverbial lighting strike. The human nervous system can rebuild and rewire itself but it is a long and fragile process. Much like a damaged electronic instrument it still works but maybe it doesn't keep good time or it just can't be relied on to perform its tasks well. This core dysfunction often becomes a vicious cycle for the addict in early recovery and this is why it takes both time and energy in a recovery atmosphere for the success to be had. A recovery community is a tolerant place of love and support that cannot be duplicated.

Fear

There is another popular expression in the recovery communities when it comes to FEAR. They have created an acronym for F.E.A.R. it goes, "F--- (f-word) Everything, And, Run," (F.E.A.R.) This is perfect for our purposes because when the addict becomes overwhelmed they will resort to their Fight or Flight limbic programming and try to escape their discomfort. They will flee the scene and take flight into their past behaviors. They will resort to the use of Freudian defense mechanisms like denial, externalization, projection, and rationalization, just to name a few.

The solution to fear is safety. Giving the newly recovering addict a safe place to heal, grow and thrive is vital to avoiding this flight back into their addictions. While "home" may seem like a good place to feel that safety it rarely works out for the better. Guilt, resentment, shame and remorse are too prevalent in the family of an addict. More complicated is the option of sending the addict off to a far away treatment program to establish their recovery. It is a quick fix but returning them home without serious reintegration into the local recovery community or a half way house is doomed to fail.

Resolving R.J.E.F.F.

The key solution to all the above stumbling blocks is quite simple. Unfortunately for the addict the solution to addiction is no more desired then the treatment for cancer: But there is only one solution that works nearly every time it is FULLY applied. Since the addicted suffer from a Mental, Physical and Spiritual/Emotional disease the solution must include all these aspects and it must be present for as long as you wish the recovery to persist. The only solutions that really work for the addicted are the 12 Step Programs of Alcoholics Anonymous, and Narcotics Anonymous. Treatment should only be seen as a route to a recovery program. Excuses kill addicts.

I would also like to warn you to avoid any current marketing ploys and snake oil salesman that tout a cure. There is no CURE for addiction and anyone who says there is, is gravely deceiving you by purposefully arranging clinical terms to argue their point and sell their program or book. Addiction is no more cured than cancer. While like cancer it can be put into remission, re-exposure to the agent that created the problem will only result in a relapse into the disease state. The best chance at success for the addict is a 12 Step Program. Why wouldn't you want to treat the problem with the best possible solution?

WHAT DO YOU DO NOW?

Having read this book is just a beginning. You can't do this alone anymore then they can. You must get help. While a professional may be able to help you sort things out, your true relief will be found in a solution similar to the alcoholic/addict, a solution that addresses both the Spiritual and Emotional.

PLEASE

Please try at least 6 different meeting locations of Al-Anon, Nar-Anon, or Adult Children of Alcoholics (ACOA.) There are no better solutions or tools for the loved one of an alcoholic/addict; they are wonderful programs. I'm sure there is a meeting near you tonight or tomorrow.

While many people in roles like mine have helped many of our clients gain clarity, the core of any successful recovery program lies in a psycho-spiritual solution, which can be adopted as a new way of living and thinking. Add to that a source of unconditional love and caring support. Meditate, do Yoga, attend church or temple, de-emphasize the addict in your daily life. Take your mind and body to a place where you can find peace so that you can gain a clear vision of the problem. Loving an alcoholic or addict creates an emotional stain on the heart and soul. I have never seen it completely removed. Stop reacting and start acting, start living your life as if. Try to live your life as if there were no addiction issue in your family. Stop insulating the addict from the consequences of their choices and their substance use. Learn to focus on meeting your own needs from the inside out, not from the outside in.

And finally, because I know the message is hard to hear:
GO TO A MEETING!!!!

Credits and References

Influential People in the Development of My Perspectives and Insights

Raymond S. John
(My father, a very loving man with an insidious disease)

Victoria Witkowski
(For her pure love and undying encouragement)

William S. Roden
(For his selfless acts to help save my soul)

Virginia Edleman and Pamela Rogan
(For their lessons in unconditional love)

Joyce Luciano
(My friend, my mentor and my soul mother)

Patricia Quinn-Stabile
(A great supervisor with a tireless commitment to helping addicts)

John M. T. Finney the 3rd
(My personal spiritual guide for keeping things simple)

Influential Perspectives in My Professional/Clinical Development

Al-Anon (1986). *"Al-Anon family groups,"* (formerly; Living with an alcoholic.) New York, Al-Anon Family Group Headquarters.

Al-Anon (1997). *"Paths to recovery; al-anon steps and traditions.,"* New York, Al-Anon Family Group Headquarters.

Al-Anon (1995). *"How Al-anon works: for families and friends of alcoholics.,"* New York, Al-Anon Family Group Headquarters.

Alcoholics Anonymous (1976) *"Alcoholics anonymous,* 3rd ED., New York, Alcoholics Anonymous World Services.

American Psychiatric Association. (2000). *"Diagnostic and statistical manual of mental Disorders.,"* (4th ed., text rev.). Washington, DC.

Barnes, A. (1998*). "Seeing through self-deception.,"* Cambridge, Cambridge University Press.

Frankl, V. (1984*). "A Man's search for meaning; an introduction to logotherapy.,"* New York : Simon & Schuster

Freud, S. (1914). *"The psychopathology of everyday life.,"* (A. A. Brill, Trans.). London: T.Fisher Unwin. (Original work published 1901).

Goffman. E (1959*) "The Presentation of self in everyday life,."* Garden City, Doubleday Anchor

Gorski, T. & Miller, M. (1982*) "Counseling for relapse prevention,"* Independence., Herald House Independence Press

Joe and Charlie (2001-11). Alcoholics Anonymous Big Book

Seminar Boca Raton Florida 2001.,
magncent7777@yahoo.com

Maslow, A (1943). "A Theory of human motivation.
Psychological Review.," New York, Harper Collins.

Maslow, A (1943) *Motivation and personality, 2nd Ed.*," New
York, Harper and Row.

McMillan, S., Rodger, R. (1996-99) For their work on the
Chronic Disease Model Education materials at Right
Turn of Maryland. (The timeline concept addiction
treatment from their client education materials
developed during their time at Right Turn of Maryland.
Owings Mills, No references sited on those materials.

Narcotics Anonymous (1988). *"Narcotics anonymous, 5th Ed.,"*
Van Nuys, World Service Office.

Peck, M. S., (1978). *"The road less traveled; A new psychology
of love, traditional values and spiritual growth.,"* New
York, Simon and Schuster.

Wilson, W. G., (1939-76). "Alcoholics anonymous, 1st & 3rd
ED.," New York, Alcoholics Anonymous World
Services.

The list of references above is generalized and knowingly vague. To be honest I have read very little on the subject of addiction (other than issues of physiology) in the last 10 years as I did not want to contaminate my own research and theories on the subject. I have attended hundreds of training with thousands of teachers. I am not a mega trainer. I work with clients and families, many more families than most of the writers you will see on the circuits today.

I have been working on this book and its content for more than 20 years and I wanted; *"Addiction; Why They Use"* to maintain its simple yet clear approach so that the layperson might better grasp this vital subject matter. I started teaching the information contained in this book as part of a community education series conducted 2 times a year starting in 2001.

However; I did feel it important to share with you, some names of the people whose perspectives have influenced my own personal learning process as these people have much to contribute towards many of the solutions we all seek. Professionals in the addiction field have always put the addict first. My priority is their families, your family, first; a people before personalities approach. I encourage you to buy your alcoholic or addict a copy of ADDICTION: Am I Powerless? (Self assessing, a user's guide to the truth). I wrote it for you, in order to get them to see what you have always wanted them to see. The truth!

In gratitude
Emmanuel S. John

May you suffer less!

www.ingramcontent.com/pod-product-compliance
Lightning Source LLC
Chambersburg PA
CBHW072240270326
41930CB00010B/2202